GW00701920

Star Doctor

By the same author

Ronald Scott Thorn

Star Doctor

Not Merely Medical Memoirs

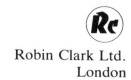

Robin Clark Ltd.
London

First published in Great Britain 1984
by Robin Clark Ltd.
A member of the Namara Group
27/29 Goodge Street, London W1P 1FD

British Library Cataloguing in Publication Data

Thorn, Ronald Scott
  Star doctor.
  1. Thorn, Ronald Scott   1. Physicians—California—
  Biography
  I. Title
  610′.92′4   R173.T/

ISBN 0-86072-074-8

Typeset by MC Typeset, Chatham, Kent
Printed and bound in Great Britain
by Mackays of Chatham Ltd, Kent

Acknowledgements

The author wishes to thank Mrs Terry Walters for typing and retyping the script and Judith Obeng and Susan Corcoran for research and additional secretarial help, and his wife for continuous encouragement. He is grateful to Roger Frisby, QC for vetting the script from the legal aspect.

He is indebted to Weidenfeld and Nicolson for permission to use quotations from *The Noël Coward Diaries* and to Hamish Hamilton for permission to quote from the biography of *Malcolm Sargent* by Charles Reid, and to the Chartered Insurance Institute of London.

And the stars . . . for being who they are.

To
MY WIFE MURIEL
With Love

Disclaimer

All the characters in this book are or were actual persons. All the incidents actually happened. All the dialogue was actually spoken. This is how I remember it. It is certainly how I like to remember it.

No attempt has been made at total recall, but since time is unhooked by memory, strict chronology has not been followed. Yet, a narrative pattern can perhaps be perceived which should make this account something more than a doctor's diary. There are no confidential medical details or secrets uncovered here. The information is locked safely in my head and in my private records. None of those mentioned is a patient of mine.

Many autobiographies are written to extol an achievement, promote a theory, or to illuminate a philosophy of life. No such pretensions are exhibited in this record. It is primarily a tale for entertainment, not posterity.

Contents

'The stars are enormous and very bright and infinity is going on all round.'

'Great big glamorous stars can be very tiresome.'

'It is sad that actors should be so consistently idiotic.'

'Really, people are *very* peculiar.'

'Life goes on and little bits of us get lost.'

'It is *still* a pretty exciting thing to be English.'

'I really must write some more when I have time.'

From *The Noel Coward Diaries*
Edited by Graham Payne & Sheridan Morley
Published by Weidenfeld & Nicolson

Foreword

Ronnie Scott Thorn and I first met as schoolboys. My father was Principal of Leicester University College and his the headmaster of a local grammar school – at which I was not a pupil. Had that been the case, and since I was a somewhat dismal scholar, I would undoubtedly now be able to boast a posterior with the unique distinction of receiving the attentions, though in opposing causes, of both father and son.

Ronnie and I met again in the fifties in London when he was writing for the stage and I was playing on it. One of his plays was mounted briefly at the Ambassadors Theatre just before my wife and I opened there in *The Mousetrap*. 'It won't run,' Ronnie diagnosed on our first night. Since it is still running and shows every sign of continuing, it is comforting to know that Ronnie now confines his prognostications to me as a patient rather than as a player.

In 1955 I was being considered for a part in a film called *The Baby and the Battleship* with my friends Johnnie Mills and Bryan Forbes. Ronnie conducted my medical. Since then he has examined me, for insurance purposes, on eighteen different occasions – the last being in 1980 just before I embarked on producing and directing *Gandhi*.

'Don't call us, we'll call you,' may be just a mildly funny catchphrase to most people but to actors and actresses, knees knocking after an interview, a reading or even a full-blown screen test, it is a nerve tingling fact of life that transforms their silent phones into objects of sheer torture. However, more often than not, the right answer, when it comes, is not a call from your agent or even the producer and director concerned. The positive answer, the one you've been praying for night and day comes, infallibly, with a call from Ronnie's admirable secretary, Judith Obeng, requesting you to make an appointment for your medical. When that happens you know, without a shadow of a doubt, that you have been cast.

Of course, it is not solely for this reason that Ronnie is held in such high esteem by people who work in the film industry. As those who read what follows will discover, he is not only wonderfully amusing company but has a truly astonishing ability to walk the tightrope between tact and discretion. To mix medicine with the mad world of movies and come up with such fizzing entertainment as this is a tonic indeed.

Sir Richard Attenborough

Star Doctor

1 Establishing Shot

Like most average boys of thirteen, in the era of the 'Hollywood Greats', the thirties, I was incorrigibly film-struck. At eye level on the wall by my bed were stuck a select row of pin ups – Marlene Dietrich, Joan Crawford, Claudette Colbert and Bette Davis. Though by then it had been decided that I was to be a doctor, I could hardly have guessed that in the not too distant future I should be asking these photographic idols in glamorous clothes to take them off; even less that I should be paid for the privilege.

At parties women are the arch interrogators. The opening lines hardly ever vary.

'Did I hear someone say you're a doctor?' American accent, husky, suntan, California.

'I have no patients.'

'You mean you're not a doctor of medicine?'

'No, what I meant . . .'

'Philosophy . . . Music?'

'I'm a Bachelor . . .'

'But . . . isn't that your wife over there?'

'Yes . . .'

'I don't get it.'

'Bachelor of Medicine.'

'Ah . . .'

'And Surgery.'

'Oh yes, I've heard about this British thing. So you're a Mister! You're a surgeon?'

'I don't ever operate.'

'Not on anyone . . .?'

'Socially perhaps,' I said with a feeble attempt at wit.

An 0.5 second pause, a brief narrowing of the lady's left palpebral fissure (for the non-technical a half-wink).

'You can say that again.'

'Socially perhaps,' I repeated obligingly.

I exchanged my questioner's empty glass of champagne for a full one from the hired waiter's passing tray. She took it and smiled.

Green eyes, ash blonde, face-lift, forty-seven passing for thirty-five. A well-preserved dish.

'OK. Let's go back to the beginning.'

'That's never possible.'

'Well, you must have some kind of specialty.'

'Yes. Insurance and Medico-legal.'

'You mean you examine murder victims . . . women who have been raped?' Definite widening of both palpebral fissures.

'No. That's forensic medicine.'

A polite champagne burp, a chuckle, a wide smile of dental perfection.

'Say, why don't you just tell me in simple words, for God's sake, just how you make a living? Where's your office for instance?'

'Consulting room.'

It was a conversation I have had many times.

The medical area of London is bounded by Marylebone Road, Marylebone High Street, Wigmore Street and Portland Place. This famous rectangle has been dubbed on TV 'The Human Jungle'. Cab drivers, more laconically, call it Pill Island. It is owned partly by the Crown, but mainly by the Howard de Walden family. The entire scene has little to do with the National Health Service, its flavour being essentially international. It boasts a number of private hospitals including the London Clinic and the famed King Edward VII Hospital for Officers (and members of the Royal Family).

Most of the buildings are occupied in the daytime by thousands of doctors, surgeons, dentists and medical auxiliaries, and also by numerous quacks, osteopaths, chiropractors, acupuncture boys, sex therapists, faith healers and some pure confidence tricksters. Every day these gentlemen – and ladies – are going quietly but intensively about their business, which is to earn private fees for their services. Everyone is very busy indeed, but it is not true that if a traffic accident occurs, or someone calls out in the street desperately 'Doctor' the only response is the sound of closing windows and slamming doors.

Behind most of the stucco façades of the buildings, the very best medical and surgical activities are being efficiently practised and the most up to date opinions expressed. Inevitably these can be conflicting. 'You pays your money and you takes your choice.'

You certainly pays your money. The large fees have to offset the astronomical rents, the very high rates, and the ineradicable British conviction that an address is a guarantee of success, if not quality, far outweighing any academic or clinical qualifications. The general practitioner in East Finchley who rents a third floor back room in the Street for half a day on Wednesdays gains a heading for his notepaper that can quadruple his normal private fees.

Nearly all the streets are one way, the main artery so to speak, Harley Street – the '*Strasse*' – running North-South, and the main vein, Wimpole Street, running parallel in the opposite direction. The pavements are beset with parking meters beside which Rolls-Royces and Mercedes nuzzle bumper to bumper. All types of clothes, robes and other gear are sported by patients walking up and down, puzzling over the confusing house numbering system. So worldwide is the quest for healing that all languages, including occasionally English, can be caught in snatches of conversation at every corner.

The area abounds in famous historical and modern references. Florence Nightingale opened her hospital at 90 Harley Street before lighting her lamp in the Crimea. Mr. Barrett practised sado-masochism on his daughter Elizabeth at 50 Wimpole Street. Thomas Hardwick built a church at the top end, and Epstein sculpted an exquisite Madonna and Child for the Convent of the Holy Child Jesus at the bottom. Gibbon wrote his *Decline and Fall* on the North side of Bentinck Street, and Arthur Wing Pinero wrote plays in Devonshire Street. Berlioz composed a few arias in Queen Anne Street, and for all I know the scientist Young enunciated his Modulus behind the blue plaque in Welbeck Street. The Germans dropped a few bombs about the place, and Christine Keeler ruined a minister of the Crown and possibly brought down a government behind curtains in a flat at 17 Wimpole Mews.

Having voted 'No' to the BMA's circulars about joining the National Health Service, I moved into the area four years after I qualified with an Oxford degree, and have been there ever since.

2 Scene One: Take One

The film and theatrical side of my practice very nearly didn't happen. One autumn day in 1948 I came home and parked my father's (borrowed) 1937 Hillman Minx without difficulty outside 38 Weymouth Street, where I occupied the ground floor and basement for both living and working.

'Any calls?' I asked Mary Eadie, the first secretary I could afford to employ.

'Yes, doctor,' she replied, I thought a little breathlessly. 'The Prudential City Office just rang to see if you could examine five artistes for "film producers' indemnity".'

'Ah, good,' I said.

'*All* this afternoon . . .!' Her eyebrows arched alarmingly.

'Excellent. But why the rush?'

'Apparently they begin shooting tomorrow!' She made it sound as if some of them would be casualties.

'You already have three consultations. I said I couldn't possibly fit them in.'

I was aghast.

'Of course you can fit them in. I'm trying to build up a practice. Apologize. Delay. Postpone. Shift people around. Make spaces.'

She made a face instead, so I added with a totally insincere smile:

'You know you're marvellous at making fa . . . spaces Mary.'

I hadn't won yet.

'But the fee quoted for each examination was only a guinea, doctor . . .'

'All right, that's five guineas, sweetie. Your salary for nearly a week. Get the Pru back on the phone and say I'll see them, there's a good girl.'

So she did. And that was the beginning.

During thousands of examinations of actors and actresses spanning a professional lifetime, I have frequently tried to detect any clinical features unique to this section of the community which distinguished it from other groups such as politicians, business men, the police or manual labourers. My general impression is that there are none; except perhaps in their mental attitude to illness or injury. The actor's determination to be fit, and to be seen to be fit under the constant glare of the public eye undoubtedly demonstrates the psychological power of mind over matter. Neurotics there may be, but there are no malingerers beyond the footlights or in front of the cameras. The cliché of 'The Show must go on' is a real force in combating organic disease in perhaps this most highly competitive of all occupations. Economics, the baleful virus which infects human beings from Los Angeles to Moscow is probably the *vis a tergo*. I understand that at any moment of time ninety-five per cent of performing artistes are not working – resting as the euphemism has it – which must just exceed the percentage of authors. I once thought of selecting certain medical parameters gleaned from my extensive records, and asking the great god Computer for an answer. But the reply would almost certainly end up in interminably boring sheets of figures. My inclination has been to stick to the far more interesting anatomical variety.

The first film actor I examined was Jack Hawkins. Over twenty years he came many times to be certified, so to speak, as medically fit to perform his roles. These became ever more important as he developed into an international star. Alas, they were later cut down to small parts when he tragically developed a gastric phonation, which removed all intonation from his very fine speaking voice. But he managed to master this method of communication, courageously overcoming his dire affliction.

I suppose Jack was the epitome of the officer and gentleman both in the parts he played and in his private life. Certainly at that first visit his character showed itself in an exemplary manner.

On that memorable day in the autumn all those years ago, Mary ushered him to the top of the stairs leading down to a London basement, where my consulting room was at that time sited.

'Good afternoon,' he said amiably, and then due to a loose stair-rod, fell down the whole flight, landing at my feet. Before I could help him, let alone administer first aid, he was up in a flash, dusted off his trousers, and adjusted his tie. He gave me a steely grin, and an even more steel-like handshake.

'I'm most terribly sorry, are you hurt?' I apologized inadequately.

'Think nothing of it, my dear doctor,' he replied. 'Entirely my clumsiness. I do hope I haven't damaged your stair-carpet.'

When I later tested his hands for a non-existent tremor I noticed that mine were shaking visibly.

My nervousness had barely died down when the next artiste arrived. I made sure there was no repetition of the Hawkins catastrophe by holding Greta Gynt's elbow as she trod elegantly in high heels down every step.

Doctors are supposed to be impervious to such things as glamour, but with young ones at any rate this is a myth. The previous tremor returned to my hands when, on request, with a disconcerting and amused stare, Miss Gynt very calmly and slowly unbuttoned the black barathea jacket of her superbly fitting costume to expose a beautifully filled filmy bra. As I listened to her heart and lungs, my professional concentration was disconcerted by an unusual noise. It was the staccato sound – rather like a short burst of automatic fire – made by the end of my stethoscope as it knocked against the large crucifix which nestled securely between her breasts.

Many years later when I examined Julie Ege, a delightful natural girl, who was even more generously endowed, the end of the same stethoscope actually broke off – an early example of stress fracture. There was a silent pause of a second or two and then we were both convulsed with laughter. A sense of humour, if not of the ridiculous, is essential sometimes both on and off the consulting couch.

The clothes many of the acting profession wear for medicals are motley in the extreme. Nowadays the punk extravagances of the Sex Pistols and the bizarre haircolouring of Toyah Wilcox pass as commonplace. But the old idea of diligent cleanliness and the wearing of scrupulously clean underwear for a doctor's examination is not now always adhered to.

The English as a whole are a dirty lot. I remember one young patient who had fractured his left great toe in an industrial injury. Accompanied by his fourteen stone Cockney mother, nineteen-year-old Alfie was six foot tall but not blessed with the highest intelligence. After I had taken down his history and learned that a careless workmate had dropped a brick on his foot, I asked Alfie to take his shoes and socks off. With a beguiling smile, he began to undo his tie. This produced an immediate response from Mum by way of a box on the ear and the admonition:

'Yer shoe, not yer tie, Alfie!'

Alfie grinned happily, riding the blow with the skill of a boxer and wrenched off his left shoe and sock, to reveal a well-scrubbed foot with a swollen big toe.

'And the other one, please,' I requested.

Alfie looked questioningly at his mother.

'Go on,' she barked. 'He wants the other one orf as well.'

Alfie still hesitated.

'I have to compare the bad foot with the good foot Alfie,' I encouraged him.

Slowly Alfie removed his other shoe and sock with difficulty. The lad's right foot did not appear to have seen soap or water for some weeks. The black and white contrast was startling, and the smell made even his mother reel backwards. She pinched her nose and rolled her eyes up in histrionic emphasis.

'Pooh . . . Alfie!' she exclaimed, and delivered her son a passable imitation of a right hook to the jaw. This time Alfie, for all his size, burst into tears.

With suitable apologies from mother, I completed the examination. As I saw them out I asked her if she had any more at home like Alfie.

'Nine,' she replied, 'and he's the brightest.'

As in Alfie's case, reluctance – or the opposite – to remove garments can give some clinical insight into character. It is extraordinary how some women take modesty to the point of obstruction. The routine request to undo a couple of buttons does not take the doctor very far if there are twelve closely set mother-of-pearls on a blouse. It also often proves impossible to apply the sphygmomanometer cuff for blood pressure by trying to push up a tight sleeve well above the elbow. An air of resentment is not unusual when the problem can only be solved by the apology, 'I'm sorry but you'll have to take your dress off.'

Oddly enough, Rudolph Nureyev is a good example of an extreme case of this: he expected me to examine him while continuing to wear his belted black leather overcoat. Admittedly, it was a very cold day. His attitude was in marked contrast to the uninhibited approach of another star who arrived commendably spot on time in her limousine, and shot across the pavement into 11 Wimpole Street, sporting a full length sable over bra and panties. But that was on a hot summer's afternoon. This was only equalled by Elizabeth Taylor, who, on one of the occasions that I examined her at her house in Hampstead wore only two garments, a caftan and the celebrated diamond. But I have always believed a lady should be allowed total freedom of choice in her own bedroom in her own home.

As opposed to what they wear when not in front of the cameras, the appearance of celebrities in the flesh can often be very different from their stage or screen persona. This provides its own protection against recognition, without recourse to well-used disguises such as dark glasses (Joan Collins) or crash helmets (Sir Ralph Richardson), but can lead to embarrassing instances of mistaken identity by the doctor's assistants.

My first wife Thelma, herself frequently confused at one time with Mara Lane, was given on occasion to saying the first thing that came into her pretty head. When she met Alan Ladd for the first time his fan told him 'Oh, you're not nearly as tall as I thought you were.'

Following the long running TV series, Thelma also managed to get things mixed up by greeting Vince Edwards with the invitation, 'Do come in, Dr. Casey.'

One dark wet night my last appointment was an hour late and we had decided to have dinner. I was just carving the roast beef when the bell rang. Thelma went to the street door. Three men in raincoats, collars up, hands in pockets, trilby brims turned down, formed a sinister circle under the street light.

The nearest one squeezed out his question through a clenched jaw.

'Doctor Thorn?'

'Who is it?' asked Thelma.

'George Raft. Mind if I come in baby?'

The mob moved forward as one man. Thelma stood her ground, albeit nervously.

'All of you?' she asked.

'Any objections?' was the quick reply.

Her nerve then gave way and she backed down the hall. I reached her side and watched the rainwater from the three coats and the three hats make three pools on the two-tone Axminster. Thelma grabbed my hand.

'This man says he's . . . '

'Mr. Raft,' I cut in. 'I'm afraid my wife didn't recognize you . . . er . . . the poor light . . . '

'That's OK kid,' said George.

He removed his hands slowly from his pockets and spread out his fingers, then treated me to a broad smile.

'See? No gun Doc.'

I realized I was still clutching the carving knife.

If you are living and practising in the same flat (known as a Reside and Practice Lease), however capacious and ingeniously planned, the two functions unavoidably get fudged from time to time. This allows for mixups or even crackups on the set due largely to the antics of the numerous extras necessarily involved in the production. These consist of reception staff, secretaries, cleaning ladies, wives and in my case two daughters. If these are of the teenage variety and the period is swinging London of the sixties, the mix can be incongruous, even bizarre.

The arrival of Mitzi Gaynor and her subsequent examination was carried out against the deafening accompaniment of *South Pacific* from the stereo-system. Both of us pretended not to notice and on leaving she sweetly signed the autograph books of Amanda, eleven, and Vanessa, nine, at the end of the performance.

My secretary, pinned to a telephone call, was beaten to the door by the two children, who, before he could reach the consulting room, processed Cary Grant through a tour of the flat. This included the old nursery and the kitchen, where he appreciatively raised the lids of the pots on the cooker and announced he was certainly looking forward to dinner.

On another occasion, redecoration of the premises was about to start and the girls had been allowed to choose the colours and décor of their individual bedrooms. Not realizing that I had a late evening appointment, Vanessa danced a rapturous series of arabesques quite naked through what she thought was an empty waiting room, declaiming ecstatically 'My room is going to be the most super super room in the whole flat!' before she noticed Dirk Bogarde. He looked up, startled, but no doubt entranced from his study of an ancient number of *Punch*.

Eventually I had to put a stop to all this and hide my appointment book as things were getting out of hand. I was warned by Thelma that the girls had invited no less than a dozen selected schoolfriends round to tea to meet the Beatles. I managed to avoid the hysterical screams and yowls of delight which would undoubtedly have greeted them by arranging to examine them in the Radiologist's rooms where they were to have their chest X-Rays.

About this time I remember a friend of mine ringing me in the middle of my examination of Tommy Steele. He asked helpfully if he could answer the phone for me. He picked up the instrument and said, 'Tommy Steele speaking.'

'Oh yes,' came the reply. 'Now pull the other one, Ronnie.'

Reception staff can be exceeedingly obtuse on occasion. Not long ago one called up to my room on the intercom a trifle indignantly.

'Dr. Thorn,' she said. 'There's a patient down here who's not on your list!'

'What's his name?' I enquired.

'A Mister Oliver.'

'That's Lord Olivier, you idiot,' I said. 'Ask him to come up straight away.'

I apologized when Sir Laurence emerged from the lift, but he was laughing and had enjoyed his joke hugely.

'What's in a name?' he said, with that famous incisive intonation.

Dickie Attenborough, whom I have known since childhood and examined literally dozens of times, is also not averse to a bit of fun. Long before he received his knighthood, he purposely confused Reception on one visit by announcing that he had come to see Sir Ronald.

The Mistaken Identity Syndrome was perhaps best demons-trated by my younger daughter Vanessa, when in her late teens she answered the door bell in Lister House. Impressed by an old schoolfriend of mine, Philip Whitfield, who on a visit from Vancouver had been to dinner with us the previous evening, she flung her arms affectionately round the patient who bore a striking resemblance to him.

'Come in, come in,' she cooed. 'How nice to see you again.'

Denholm Elliott, never at a loss in any social situation, responded suitably but covered Vanessa with confusion by remarking to me 'What a charming new receptionist you have.'

As every patient knows, and if they don't they soon discover, that with the best will in the world, and the most careful appointment system, the very nature of the work unavoidably forces doctors at times to keep people waiting. I hate to do this, though I dislike rather more to be kept in a pre-coronary state myself, wondering how late someone will be, or worse, if they will turn up at all. This behaviour is a totally successful aggressive act against which one has no defence. When I am the culprit, and apologies are met with truculent complaints, I have found the best answer is to suggest serious consideration of the meaning of the word 'patient'.

In the case of film artistes, I have found that the real 'greats' – Sir Laurence, Sir John, Sir Michael and Sir Richard for example – are all meticulous about punctuality, a trait which certainly puts them at the top in my book.

While waiting, sleep is often the best escape. Comfortable seating is a great aid to this. To rouse or not to rouse and the manner of arousal is always a tricky problem. I remember George Sanders dropped off within three minutes of arrival, so I gave him half an hour's doubtless well earned kip before shaking him extremely gently.

At 3 Bentinck Mansions, as with George Raft, I had given up George Cole, who was due one day at 6.00 p.m. At 8.30, after dinner, I happened to go into the waiting room and snap on the lights. He awoke with a start from a supine position on the couch. The receptionist had gone off two hours previously without letting me know Mr. Cole had arrived. We both apologized and were very nice to each other about the situation. We still are.

This was not so embarrassing as the events which overtook a young French star, who was brought to her medical direct from Heathrow by the producer himself, who was literally propping her up at the door. We half carried her into the consulting room. A first year medical student could have diagnosed that she had consumed an overabundance of champagne all the way from Orly. I explained that it was not fair to the girl, the producer or the insurance company to attempt to examine her in the state she was in. I suggested he took her away, and brought her back early the following morning. He told me she was due to fly back to Paris in three hours' time, and implored me, insurance being essential before shooting began the next day, to let her rest for a time and could I not give her something to sober her up? Coffee was produced and shortly she was able to make a request to go to the bathroom, and what's more make the journey unaided.

10

The producer and I chatted about this and that, but after twenty minutes I became anxious that she might have fainted or even passed out. I investigated. The bathroom door was unbolted. I went inside. Mademoiselle had completely stripped and was fast asleep in the bath.

I do not know who the lady was because, as I never got to examine her, my records do not record her name.

3 Background Music

Antecedents, childhood memories, faded photographs, the early influence of characters and places, intense half-forgotten loves and passions form the background music to any autobiography. Strangely time-distant sights, sounds, smells and voices come back over the years with perfect clarity, like newly-minted etchings and unscratched 78 records.

I was born at 2.00 a.m. on 27 April, 1920 in a large brass-knobbed bedstead in the front bedroom of an Edwardian house at 23 Craven Street, Melton Mowbray in the County of Leicestershire, not very far from the geographical centre of England. I am told the labour was long and arduous. My deliverer was a Doctor Montague Dixon, MD, who sported a black jacket, striped trousers, grey spats and a monocle. A few years later he let me sit on his knee and help to steer his grey bull-nosed Morris two seater with a dickey-seat behind. I think really I wanted to become a doctor because you must have a car and drive around in it.

My father was an assistant master at the Grammar School. Although he had a BSc in economics he in fact taught mathematics, geography, English, Latin and music. He had auburn hair. My mother was a very beautiful woman who had been the secretary of Sir William Brockington, the Director of Education in Leicester. Her hair was silken, long and put up in a tight bun held by a tortoiseshell comb. Her hair was almost jet black. Mine was medium mouse and has remained so.

The most intelligent thing I ever did was to choose these two people for parents. I loved them both, worshipped my mother and adored my father. They accorded me the obsessive affection known as spoiling their only child – though the rod was not entirely spared. There has been so much psycho-analytical claptrap written about this solo situation, but I cannot recall any sense of deprivation, loneliness, pain or unhappiness during the first

11

fourteen years of my life. However I do accept the psychiatric profession's second contention, that a happy childhood moulds the spirit for life.

I did not go to school until I was seven. Before that age it seemed a superfluous exercise. My mother taught me my multiplication tables by rote, showed me via pothooks how to write copperplate in copybooks, and encouraged me to read from a small thick red-bound book called *Reading Without Tears*. She was quite strict and in fact there were a few tears. I remember now declaiming the repetitive lines of heavy type '. . . Big Beg Bag Bog Bug . . . Fig Feg (whatever that was) Fag Fog Fug . . .' My father took me in arithmetic through to long division and pounds, shillings, pence, halfpennies and farthings. He taught me the first two declensions of Latin nouns and the simple tenses of the first conjugation of verbs. He stuck a large poster-map of the world plastered with the red patches of the British Empire on the wall opposite my bed. I used to gaze at it on long light summer evenings, listening to my parents' voices and laughter coming up through the open window from the garden, where they often dined *al fresco* from a little trolley. My father bought me a Scottish Terrier puppy called Bunty, one of whose ears refused to cock up. When she died from distemper a year later my heart was broken for the first time, but cardiac muscle is surprisingly resilient. Mine has been emotionally scarred many times since, yet continues to function.

My father, Bunty and I tramped through the fields and splashed through the streams around Melton. My father was a mine of information on the countryside and natural history. He wrote verse about birds and animals for *The Field*. He had a fine light baritone voice and on Saturday afternoons, his half-day, if it was wet, I would sit on top of his flexed knees while he lay on the drawing-room couch. He would sing sea-shanties and ballads, while we consumed a quarter of a pound of Radiance toffee or Liquorice Allsorts.

Armed with this abundance of home-spun education and the ability to read Teddy Tail in the *Daily Mail* at the age of six, it was not surprising that I achieved immediate academic success when I went to Windybrow preparatory school, situated half-way up Burton Hill. At the end of my first year I received a prize for nine firsts. All the subjects in the curriculum. Admittedly, the competition was not very hot. There were only seventeen boys and girls, of which one was a cretin and another an achondroplasic dwarf. Margaret Atter, the wife of an alcoholic solicitor, ran the establishment in her own home. The school pet was a disgusting owl called 'Chippy' which used to fly in from the garden through an open window and land on one's head. Mrs. Atter and Chippy shared two remarkable resemblances; their staring eyes and musty smell. My prize was nevertheless astutely inscribed with the warning 'Ronnie must learn not to get a swollen head'. This phenomenon was certainly cut down to size years later at Shrewsbury by my gaining three per cent in my first examination in German. I was henceforth known for a time as 'Three-per-cent Thorn'.

Two other incidents remain clearly in my memory from my stay at Windybrow. One was anatomical; the beautiful silk-stockinged legs of a Miss Richardson who was the assistant mistress and all of nineteen years old. We used to have a reading class round a large mahogany dining-room table covered with a red velvet cloth whose fringes reached nearly to the floor. I developed a habit that after my turn at reading out a paragraph from E. Nesbit's *The Railway Children* (later I was to examine Jenny Agutter for the main part in Lionel Jefferies' successful film), I would slip off the bench and observe in close detail Miss 'Rich's' slender lower limbs crossing and uncrossing in the semi-darkness, keeping an ear-up the while for the reading as it proceeded round the table above, so that I could reappear in good time for my turn when it came again. If my temporary absence had been noted, I had the excuse ready that I had dropped a pencil or rubber. The game came to an abrupt end, however, when temptation overcame me and one day I gently stroked the beautiful contour of my teacher's calf. A shriek worthy of a 'Carry-On' farce occurred. I was pulled out red-faced from my lair, and sent home for the day with a suitable note. My mother feigned shock. My father gave me what is known as an old-fashioned look.

The other incident was respiratory and gastric. One of my contemporaries at Windybrow was Bruce Hobbs, who later won the Grand National on Battleship, the youngest jockey ever to do so. His father, the trainer Reg Hobbs, and his wife Margery were close friends of my parents. They lived just around the corner of Craven Street. On the occasion in question, Bruce's father had carelessly left open in the dining-room a box of Ramon Allones to which Bruce helped himself liberally. He generously offered me one of the full coronas and we sat behind the laurel bushes in the school garden and smoked at least two inches of the cigars before the inevitable reflexes took their toll.

Bruce introduced me to the world of horses and riding as also did Natty Russell, the son of a well-known groom. My parents could not afford to buy me a pony, let alone pay for its weekly upkeep. So from Bruce and Natty I learnt to ride clandestinely and was also able to borrow mounts from their stables. The first pony I was put out on constantly pulled to the left, but I was told was docile enough unless it came across a tar-barrel. I started off down a lane with Bruce who was on a superb hunter. Fifteen minutes later we encountered not just one but a whole pile of tar-barrels at a corner. Immediately the pony reared up and off I came.

Undaunted, very early one morning Natty contrived to get me out on a beautiful chestnut, a prodigious number of hands high. I seemed to be sitting on top of a walking tower. Natty instructed me vociferously from his own mount. I walked, I trotted, I cantered and then we were off on a hair-raising gallop. How I kept my seat, I shall never know but I stayed on for miles and miles until the horse came to a halt.

My parents were very worried not to find me in my bed at 8.00 a.m. They enquired of the milkman on his daily round if he had seen me.

'Oh yes,' he smiled. 'Going like the wind over Brentingby level crossing.'

I reached home an hour later with a very sore bottom but a feeling of triumph.

'Can I go hunting, next season?' I asked.

'With the Quorn or the Belvoir?' my father enquired with amusement.

'Oh I don't mind,' I said.

'Sorry boy,' he replied. 'I can't afford it. Not even the togs.'

And so I had to be content with occasional rides on borrowed ponies. That was as far as my horsemanship ever got.

It was about this time that I first went to the cinema, which was to play such an important part in my life. The picture house at Melton in the twenties was at the end of a narrow little street off the market place just round the corner from the Penny Bazaar. This embryo Marks and Sparks was a necessary call on the way to the Saturday afternoon matinée, to obtain a supply of Bulls-eye peppermints – one ounce for a halfpenny – to gobble away during the performance. I usually went with Bruce and Joan Hollingshead, the family butcher's daughter who had very blue eyes and long black pigtails tied with red ribbon bows. We paid for threepenny seats in the balcony and gazed in wonder at the flickering silent screen, the pianist pointing the action with suitable extemporization, and with a skill which I feel was far more appropriate than the early years of the 'Talkies'.

There was no such thing then as 'A', 'U' or 'X' categories and as children we were exposed to any material which the primitive Hollywood cared to churn out. The feature was often a comedy. Charlie Chaplin did not greatly amuse me, any more than he did when I examined him later in a house at Virginia Water. I found him to be a sad, withdrawn personality which some say was the secret of his genius. I much preferred the Keystone Cops and the villains of the Westerns. But the thrill of the show was always the weekly serial. This had a profound effect on me. It frightened me stiff. Those old silent black and white images were perhaps nothing like as horrific as the pictures one can see almost daily in the present children's diet of fear on TV, but at the time they were just as persuasive. The serial was called *The Spider*. Each episode ended in a gruesome murder. Before the alarming and sinister words 'To be Continued' appeared, the last close-up showed a huge spider's web pinning down the corpse with sickening inevitability.

Soon I took to waking up shortly after going to bed and crying out in alarm, convinced that on the eiderdown which covered me were the sticky strands of my own arachnid's deadly trap.

When she rushed into my bedroom to investigate my nightmare I did not tell my mother the source of my fear. I suppose because children like to be frightened as long as they are in safe familiar surroundings, and perhaps because an explanation might have precipitated the greater fear of being forbidden to go to the flicks.

A night-light in a saucer was placed by my bed, but the dancing flame projected even more frightening shapes on the ceiling and walls. An early neon light bulb was substituted but my fertile imagination turned the pink glowing coils into the bones of a skeleton. The journey to bed soon became an ordeal as I passed the blackened old oil painting of an evilly grinning cavalier which hung on the corner wall where the last four stairs turned onto the landing. I ran past it with my head down. The gilt-framed monstrosity, incidentally, was no ancestral portrait, but was purchased for five shillings in a junk-shop by my father, I suspect in the hope that it might turn out to be an early study of Franz Hals's masterpiece in the Wallace Collection. It wasn't of course and eventually the hanging cord broke and the picture fell down, interpreted as a sign of doom by my mother, who was prey to endless superstitions – broken mirrors, crossed knives, spilt salt, a fear of thunder, and the dire consquences of seeing a new moon through glass.

Eventually my father put paid to my nocturnal antics by singing me a verse of 'Golden Slumbers', then snapping out the light, closing the bedroom door firmly and leaving me in the pitch dark to sweat it out. But I'm still not very fond of spiders.

Melton Mowbray was adorned with a beautiful perpendicular parish church. I attended morning service with my parents from a very early age. On one particular Sunday I was rather excited, at the same time overawed by the intelligence that a visiting Canon Blakeney was to give the sermon. Fidgety as little boys are in such situations I repeatedly asked my father as the dignitaries in their robes solemnly paraded up the aisle, 'Is that Canon Blakeney?', only to be told that it was not.

The lessons were read. As each solemn personage performed his duty I persisted with my questioning.

'Is *that* Canon Blakeney?'

'No.'

Hymns were announced by the vicar.

'Is that Canon Blakeney?'

'No. Now be quiet.'

At last a great giant of a man weighing at least fifteen stone mounted the pulpit and gazed threateningly down on us from above the great Golden Eagle lectern.

'Is *that* Canon Blakeney?' I whispered, this time grasping my mother's hand.

'Yes,' came the answer.

My reply was equally definite.

'I want to go to the laventry.'

At that time Malcolm Sargent, my godfather, was the parish organist and had shared digs with my father before he got married. They shared also many other things, a similar sense of humour and a love of music. My father was an accomplished amateur pianist and mimic and could play any melody by ear after one hearing, and read any music from sight. In fact his natural musical talent had only been discovered because he had been sent to finish the twelfth lesson of a course started by my very much less talented Auntie Elsie, so that no money would be wasted. While Malcolm and my father were together, my father composed a ballad called 'My Heart Has a Quiet Sadness' and Sargent the professional set it to music. It was published by Chappells at two shillings and was first sung at the Queen's Hall by a celebrated English tenor of the time, John Coates. In his biography of Malcolm Sargent, Charles Reid describes the three stages of the ballad as 'modulating from the initial quiet sadness to a soul throbbing with madness and love waiting in the vale'. But I'm afraid that Eric Bloom the critic didn't share his enthusiasm, and wrote that it was 'a light and sentimental song, words by a hack writer, set to music by a composer of no merit'.

However, his opinion utterly failed to dampen the ebullience and energy of either Tom or Malcolm. They formed the Melton Amateur Operatic Society which doubled with performances at Stamford where Sargent lived for the first eighteen years of his life. Sargent conducted and my father played all the Lytton parts in every one of the Gilbert & Sullivan operas. My mother was in the chorus. Music and laughter seemed to wash through our house like a never-ending 'Rustle of Spring', but even then my own musical inclinations were to the first throbbing beats of ragtime which were coming across the Atlantic. I was introduced to it by my young Uncle Charlie, when he came over on visits from Staffordshire. He ran a jazz-band and when he took me at the age of twelve to Leicester Opera House, the full blasting magic of Louis Armstrong's first European tour left me in a daze for weeks. Thereafter, I gave up piano lessons and one of the happiest moments of my life was when my parents sent me a trumpet as a birthday present at Shrewsbury. It was a silver-plated B-flat trumpet – a special inexpensive line from Boosey & Hawkes. But that didn't matter. I was hooked. I had lessons from the OTC band tutor, Sergeant Major Addison, who first reported that my playing was weak in the upper register. He later was horrified by my unorthodoxy in deserting 'Colonel Bogey' and 'El Abenico' for 'Ain't Misbehavin', but also astounded that I was producing growls, smears, top C's with lip-trills, and bringing down the roof of the Alington Hall.

For most of the year Melton Mowbray was a sleepy market town, given to making pork pies and Stilton cheese. But from just before Christmas to the following March it was transformed into what can only be described as a rural Mayfair. The place became stocked with hunters, and also glamorous huntresses of the aristocracy. They rented houses in and around the town for the fox-hunting season with the Quorn, the Belvoir and the Cottesmore.

The effect on me was electric. At the top end of Craven Street, Baroness Ravensdale, Lord Curzon's daughter, took up residence. At the bottom Mrs. Julian Lezard – whose former husband was Mike Wardell, editor of *The Evening Standard* – rented a hunting box. The four sons of George V, Edward, Prince of Wales, Albert, Duke of York, Henry, Duke of Gloucester and George, Duke of Kent, occupied Craven Lodge halfway down Burton Hill.

Because of my father's talent as an entertainer at the piano, he was frequently asked to play and sing at after-dinner smoking parties. The favourite request of the Royals was 'I Do Like an Egg for My Tea'. Because of his outstanding ability as a natural teacher he was engaged as a tutor to bolster the flagging academic abilities of hordes of Etonians. A Rolls was sent for him to go to Belvoir Castle. A lot of the time he taught in our drawing room. Dan, the Earl of Ranfurly and later Governor of the Bahamas, Corky and Simon Wardell who was just a little older than me, all sons of the beautiful Hilda Lezard, frequently came to our house. As a natural spin-off from these activities I was invited to the numerous children's parties, most of which were quite lavish affairs. I enjoyed myself enormously and this seasonal foray of a simple country lad into the lifestyle of the upper-crust – which included sitting for a brief half minute on the future King Edward VIII's knee at Craven Lodge – produced a lack of awe of the famous and illustrious, but an awful propensity for name-dropping which stood me in good stead when settling into my film insurance practice. I don't think I ever felt any pangs of envy about the large gap between the very rich and the moderately poor, which was my own background; except for Simon's gold propelling pencil which had been inscribed to him with 'Love from Tallulah'. By the time I examined Miss Bankhead many years later, I had risen above it.

I will record, however, the occasion when two of the Royal Dukes, I can't recall which, were walking down Craven Street from the stables after an early morning ride. No doubt the foggy midland air caused one of them to hawk and spit over our front garden privet hedge. My father, who was shaving at the open bathroom window above, observed the act without comment. It was the following summer when we were on a family seaside holiday at Hunstanton in Norfolk and had joined a sight-seeing day-trip, that he returned the compliment through the beautiful wrought iron gates of Sandringham.

4 Script Conference

The questions which have to be put to the artiste vary in number and content according to the insurer who is indemnifying the film production company. The doctor's job is to point out the likelihood of loss due to illness of the actors while the film is being made.

In assessing these medical risks, those conditions which are long-term, though potentially serious, can be disregarded. Overweight or mild hypertension in the relatively young, a family history of stroke or controlled diabetes become irrelevant in the short term. As little as four weeks can be the time it takes to make a picture nowadays. By contrast minor conditions such as recurrent styes of the eyelids or Herpes Simplex of the lips or severe hay-fever could pose a problem with close-up photography.

The medical examiner can recommend an exclusion of any particular condition from the policy. (Only on three occasions in thousands of examinations have I stated a person to be uninsurable.) It may sound a callous outlook but if life expectation is below average, the film underwriter is not really interested. As long as the artiste lasts to the end of shooting, he can drop dead the next day and no one seems to care other than to give a sigh of relief. Pregnancy, alcoholism or drug-taking are in most instances automatically excluded.

Failure of the artiste to disclose to the doctor any relevant information can lead to the policy being repudiated.

Should an illness interrupt shooting – with the daily loss of thousands of dollars – which might have been avoided had the true medical history been mentioned, unhappy and acrimonious disputes may occur. This situation is surprisingly rare. Excuses from the artistes about past illnesses such as 'I forgot', or 'I didn't think it was important', or 'But it was such a long time ago', cut little ice with the claims assessors and loss adjusters. Though insurers are in the risk business, the last thing they want to take is a risk. This attitude I strongly defend, since otherwise there would be little need for medical examinations.

As they get older artistes are tempted to lie about their true age. It is a useless ploy because back records can always be consulted. On one or two occasions I have noted that certain individuals seem to be getting younger. Very rarely is the answer given to the question 'Are you perfectly well and in sound health?' other than a resounding affirmative. The response can be more dramatic. Peter Sellers once terrified me by way of reply to this question by getting up from his chair and standing on his head. Spike Milligan's instant retort was 'It's a lie! Who said that?'

In the questionnaire is a long list of various conditions which have to be put to the patient individually. Noel Coward's ever present wit demolished the tedium of this catechism with brilliant despatch. In order to savour the full effect of his reply it is necessary to realize that all his answers were given very seriously, without any facial expression, or a second's hesitation and in the same tone of voice using a slightly rising inflection. The result came out as follows:

'Mr. Coward, have you ever had or suffered from fits? . . .'
'No.'
'Heart disease?'
'No.'
'Hypertension?'
'No.'
'Cerebro-vascular accident?'
'No.'
'Disease of the kidneys, urinary tract or bladder?'
'No.'
'V.D?'
'Constantly.'

The demonstrable untruth of this answer was the essence of its humour.

Another question was neatly turned by Victor Mature. I should have expected something of the sort because like everyone else I had heard the story that when he had been asked to fight a lion in one biblical epic, he refused point-blank.

'No come on, Vic, the animal's been drugged,' said the director soothingly.

'Yeah . . .?'

'He's a very old lion.'

'Yeah . . .?'

'Hell, we've drawn all his teeth, Vic!'

'So who wants to be gummed to death?'

My question was much more innocent.

'Mr. Mature, have you in the last twenty-one days been exposed to any infectious or contagious disease?'

Vic pondered the question seriously for several seconds. The reply came equally seriously.

'Now let's see . . . Monday it was Doris, Tuesday it was Marigold, Wednesday it was . . .' and so on. The joke was certainly on me.

A question which appears on some of the forms can provoke a surprising reaction. Many years ago Orson Welles was in London to make a film, and as is so often the case the insurance medical somehow gets left to the last minute, or even until after the first day's shooting. I was asked to see Mr. Welles at 7.00 p.m. at the Dorchester. Things had apparently not gone too well at the studios, and the great man was in a tetchy mood. I was greeted outside his suite by the producer, the co-producer and the director and apprised of this fact. I went into the bedroom. Mr. Welles was resting on his bed. The questions were duly asked and answered without incident until I put the one about previous pictures.

'State the titles of the last three films in which you have taken part.'

'Why do I have to answer that?' snapped Orson irritably.

'So that they can look up your previous insurances,' I replied.

'It's none of their business.'

'All right,' I said. 'If you like, I'll just put "Artiste declined to answer".'

'Don't be insolent,' he growled.

'No insolence intended, but I do have to put the question.'

There was a full half-minute's silence. Then, in that magnificent deep sonorous voice, the replies came out impressively.

'*Macbeth.*'

'*Macbeth*,' I wrote down.
'*Othello*.'
'*Othello*,' I repeated.
Then all hell broke loose.
'I will not go on with this charade,' he barked at me. 'I refuse absolutely to answer these tom-fool questions. Now get out. Go on, get out.'

When someone as large as Orson Welles roars an order with the full force of his talented ability, it takes a braver man than me to refuse to obey it. I got out with as much dignity as there was time for.

When I closed the door behind me, the assembled company had obviously heard the outburst. An air of urgent tension pervaded the atmosphere.

'What happened?' I was asked anxiously. 'Has he passed for insurance?'

'I haven't examined him.'

'Why not? What have you been doing in there?'

'Trying to get him to answer certain questions. He refused.'

'Hell!' said the director.

'But he *has* to be insured,' exclaimed the producer. 'Now don't go doctor. I know how to handle this. Can you wait awhile?'

'Very well,' I said, looking at my watch, 'but don't make it too long.'

To my surprise he shook me by the hand, and drawing himself up as they say disappeared through the door.

There followed an altercation of some considerable heat and volume. Odd phrases and words got through to us.

'. . . Gestapo! I will not be subjected to this!' and so forth. Eventually things became quieter and the producer finally emerged looking as though he had been mauled by Victor Mature's lion. I was again shaken by the hand. A decidedly moister encounter.

'He'll see you now. It'll be OK now,' was the reassurance. 'I promise you Doc. Thanks for waiting. These great guys can be very temperamental. I guess that's why they're great. Go in now. Thanks Doc. We've just *got* to get him insured. You understand that?'

'I understand,' I said feebly and eased my way back into the lion's den.

The scene couldn't have been more different, the atmosphere more congenial. Mr. Welles was now wearing a dressing-gown which Noel would not have spurned, and was sitting in one of the Dorchester reproduction bergères.

'Come in doctor, come in,' he said affably. 'Sit down. What would you like, Scotch on the rocks or a Bourbon?' He poured me a drink. 'Cigarette? Here take the pack.'

I accepted his offers and sat opposite him.

'I guess,' he growled fruitily, 'I owe you an apology.'

'Not at all,' I said, succumbing to his overwhelming charm. 'We all have off days.'

'You can say that again. And have I had an off day! That Studio is full of cretins. Little more ice?'

'No thank you.'

'OK. Now this medical. Shoot.'

I took out the form and my biro.

'Well, we reached the point where your last two pictures were *Macbeth* and *Othello*. I just want one more.'

I had a fleeting sensation that everything was going to explode again. In a way it did. The mobile features dissolved into a totally disarming smile, and then as the great torrent of laughter burst out the huge body shook with Falstaffian mirth.

'The third and last picture I made, my dear doctor, was called . . .' His amusement became uncontrollable and tears streamed down his face.

'. . . was called *Getting Gertie's Garter*,' he finally got out.

I wrote the title down solemnly. Then the infectous laughter overcame me.

'No wonder, Mr. Welles,' I said, 'you didn't want to say that.'

'Hell,' he gurgled, 'of course not. You're perceptive.' He smiled conspiratorially. 'But you know once in a while – one has to make these B pictures – a guy has to make a living.'

The remainder of the medical passed off in a frankly convivial atmosphere.

Years later when the great 'Duke' towered into my consulting room, he impressed me with the sheer size of his personality. John Wayne sat in the chair by my desk and pre-empted nearly all my quetions at the outset.

'Doc,' he said, 'sitting in this chair of yours is just about the fittest person you're ever likely to examine.' There seemed little I could advance as a contrary argument. 'I am the man,' he said, 'who's beaten the big "C".'

Tragically he was dead in two years.

A similar near-tragedy I encountered some years earlier. In fact it was the occasion of a new question appearing thereafter on certain insurance company forms: 'Are you prepared to accept any reasonable treatment prescribed by the insurer's medical advisers?'

A young and beautiful actress contracted lobar pneumonia in the middle of a picture. Her own doctor was a foreign gentleman who practised a strange mixture of herbalism and faith healing. He had a very persuasive personality and was charming in the extreme, which no doubt explained his success in building up a sizeable practice amongst the acting profession. In passing, it has often been said that the most unorthodox medical treatment has always been enthusiastically favoured by the top and bottom of the social scale. At the turn of the century when black coats, button-holes and striped trousers were *de rigueur* in Harley Street, it was unkindly observed that the number of silver-framed signed photographs of the illustrious on show in a consulting room was inversely proportional to the skill of the incumbent.

The lady of this story became very ill indeed. Having qualified after the era of chemotherapy and during the advent of antibiotics, I had never seen an actual clinical case of pneumonia go through its alarming stages of white hepatization, red hepatization and crisis with its unfortunate proportion of fatalities. The patient and her husband had absolute faith in their doctor. Mine was tempered with reservations when I learnt that his treatment consisted *inter alia* of sprinkling Lycopodium powder on the patient's abdomen.

As the lady's condition deteriorated I called in an eminent consultant physician from a well-known chest hospital. We were faced with a brick wall. My colleague pulled no punches in describing the dire consequences which might ensue unless admission to hospital or at least an immediate recourse to antibiotics was not followed. After an hour or more of fruitless persuasion, we had to give up and retired sad and defeated. The upshot was a long illness, and an enormous claim which was followed by eventual recovery – a tribute to the natural processes of resistance of the human body. The illogical conclusion of the patient and her husband was 'You see? We knew she would get better if we followed our doctor's instructions.' As they forked out, the insurance company's reaction was not so complacent.

The light shed on a person at a medical examination arises not only from the patient. Interesting and illuminating clues are provided by what or whom they bring with them. Zsa Zsa Gabor arrived with a dog and a maid, two days late at an unscheduled appointment.

'My doggie has a very nasty cough,' she announced.

'Would you listen to him first please, darlink,' she begged me charmingly.

Unnecessarily pompously I told her doggies were not in my field, which remark made her pout characteristically. To soften the blow I added, 'But I have a cousin who is a highly qualified vet in Leicestershire. I could let you have his 'phone number.' I don't remember the breed in question, but her pet snuffled and sneezed close by throughout my painstaking examination of the sounds made by his mistress's flawless bronchial tree.

Judy Geeson also usually brings a dog to a medical but both are so well behaved that there has never been any tangle of dog-leads and stethoscope tubes. David Attenborough is exceedingly circumspect but I always feel he may have a salamander in his pocket. James Mason brings his wife, and Anita Ekberg brought one of her husbands, Anthony Steele, who, for reasons best known to himself, insisted on accompanying me behind the screen while I examined her. Diana Dors once brought her leg in a plaster-cast, Edward Fox brought a spare pair of trousers – on their way to the cleaners, and of course Richard Burton brought a mink coat. But the nicest thing for me was brought as a gift by Nigel Davenport. Reputed to be Jomo Kenyatta's original flyswitch carried back from a film location in Africa, it hangs permanently in my waiting room, its carved hardwood native-head handle reassuring those patients nowadays who swear by witchdoctors.

5 Tracking Shot

In 1929 we moved from Melton Mowbray to Barrow-on-Soar, a large village four miles from Loughborough. My father had been appointed headmaster, the youngest in the area, of an old county grammar school. It was founded in 1717 by Humphrey Perkins, one-time Chaplain Extraordinary to Charles II. As a result the school had a magnificent crest of an eagle on argent and the motto '*Honeste Audax*'. The previous headmaster, who had stayed for three years, had exuded a general flamboyance in the endless dinner parties he gave and the ways he raised funds for the school. In keeping with his character, he had insisted the motto should be translated as 'Nobly Daring' but my father changed it back to the more prosaic 'Honourably Brave'. My father's predecessor's ways had not endeared him to the rather suspicious local inhabitants and the rural community from which the school drew its girl and boy pupils. When first introduced as the new headmaster to the Chairman of the Governors, my father was greeted with a baleful glare and the unnerving comment 'Well, I hope you're a better bugger than the last one.'

But to me the move was an exciting expansion of activities. To live in the School House through every holiday may not have sounded attractive to many boys – indeed my second cousin John Fox when asked if he wanted to come to Humphrey Perkins as a boarder with Uncle Tom replied lugubriously 'No thanks. Algebra for breakfast and geometry for tea.' Nevertheless, he duly came, as did also his younger brother Roger, now a successful vet in Market Harborough, the person to whom I recommended Zsa Zsa Gabor to take her doggie.

At the end of every term as soon as I had said goodbye to my form-mates, I indulged to the full the variety of amenities which were mine for the asking: the playing fields, the gymnasium, the laboratories where I manufactured stink bombs and fireworks. I asked friends to play tennis and badminton, and read avidly a large quantity of books in the reference library. I conversed with old Langton the caretaker amid the acrid fumes of the stokehole, and climbed over the forbidden many-gabled roofs. I roller-skated round the corridors, kicked a football up into the ancient walnut tree to bring down the nuts and helped myself without stint to the fruits of a well-stocked kitchen garden, and orchard – to the extent that one afternoon, sent to pick raspberries for my mother's jam-making, I consumed one for every two picked. This led to several hours of non-stop vomiting during the night. For many years my prayers ended thus '. . . for Thine is the Kingdom the Power and the Glory, and please God don't let me be sick tonight'.

Having been given a bicycle I sped round the village making a general nuisance of myself with indefatigable questioning of shopkeepers, the butcher, the baker, the chemist, the postmistress, and notably the builders, Ball Sons and Squires, who attended to the repairs and maintenance at the school. Tom Squires, a lay preacher of no mean vigour, also doubled as the village undertaker. He mainly passed the time regaling me with tales of the trenches; but one day, when I was being particularly tiresome in his workshop and incidentally had ruined a chisel, a spokeshave and a plane, he decided to teach me a lesson.

'All right Master Ronald, I think it's time we buried you. Say your prayers.' He and his assistant Wilf caught me after a brief chase round the benches, lifted me struggling and shouting and then placed me in a newly made coffin and put on the lid.

'Screw him up, Wilf.' I heard the muffled command through the musty smelling elmwood of what I was now convinced was my last resting place.

'Straight to the church, Tom?' I heard Wilf enquire.

'That's right Wilf,' was the reply. 'There's a nice grave just been dug behind the vestry!'

I kicked and bellowed as I felt my wooden overcoat being lifted and carried along. Of course they let me out a few seconds later. I cycled home faster than I had ever done before. On reflection the experience refuted yet another of the psychiatrists' dicta; I have never been subject to claustrophobia.

During these years my hobbies and interests narrowed their field from Hornby trains, meccano, and the inevitable stamp, cigarette-card and birds' egg collecting, kite flying, and model aircraft making to the more exacting pursuits of entomology, watercolour drawing, cinema-going and girls.

Jack Tatham, who was a few years older, had a magnificent collection of butterflies and moths largely bequeathed to him by his father who had been a serious lepidopterist all his life.

Jack and I roamed the beautiful countryside of Charnwood Forest and Bradgate Park on expeditions, armed with apparatus obtained from Watkins & Doncaster (six doors from Charing Cross), nets, poison bottles, little glass-bottomed boxes for taking caterpillars, pupae and even clusters of tiny eggs laid on the underside of leaves. We also took slabs of Rowntree's motoring chocolate and bottles of Tizer for provisions. It was serious work.

Having read White's *Selbourne* I had vivid fantasies of becoming a celebrated naturalist, a strange omen for the future when I went to Shrewsbury to discover Charles Darwin was perhaps its most celebrated pupil. Moths were in a way more fascinating than the butterflies, not least because their collection gave a watertight excuse for staying up late.

I kept a detailed notebook of observations like all good students of natural history. I can recall now the excitement of going round the 'sugar' patches painted on tree-trunks, posts and palings at dusk to lay the sticky bait, and two hours later visiting the same areas with a torch often to find hordes of specimens guzzling away. Intoxicated, they were easily coaxed into boxes or the killing bottle ready for 'setting' the next day.

Glancing through the pages of my diary written in round half-formed juvenile lettering I came across some solemn entries.

'*General Notes for 1933.* I did not rear any caterpillars during 1933. The season was a good one. I have now a good recipe for "Sugar".

28⅓% Stale Beer
28⅓% Black Treacle
28⅓% Brown Sugar
15% English Honey

Heat until in a liquid state thin enough to be painted with a brush.'

Of course half the attraction of the game lay in the magic of the names like The Flounced Rustic (*Luperina tertacea*); The Hebrew Character (*Noctua C-Nigrum*); The Pebble Hook-tip (*Drepona falcataria*); The Hart and Dart (*Agrotis exclamationes*) and the celebrated Painted Lady (*Vanessa cardui*).

The residue of all this intense activity now hangs in a decorative column of glass-fronted cabinet drawers on a wall in my waiting room in Harley Street. They often form brief topics of conversation which put nervous patients at their ease. I pass suitable comments but make no profound observations. I ceased making those at the age of four.

In the holidays, there was a small number of children who became my regular companions. Donald Thomas, the vicar's son, Jack Tatham, Marie and Eva Gray, the daughters of the village G.P., a humorous diminutive Scotsman married to a saucer-eyed French lady from Lyon, who never completely mastered English and ended most sentences with her translation of the French '*n'est pas?*' as 'in't it?' There was also Shirley and Phillipa Hardy-Smith and Gurth Holland. We all met at each others' homes frequently.

At Donald Thomas's eleventh birthday party 'Sardines' was decided upon as the opening frolic before tea consisting of bread and butter, scones and strawberry jam, cucumber sandwiches, cream buns, biscuits and various highly-coloured jellies. Donald elected to become 'It' and disappeared to hide. After five minutes we all searched the rambling vicarage to find him. The object of the exercise was, once found, to stay with the person hiding until the end of the game. Then, when everyone was crammed into some stuffy cupboard silent as church mice, the last one to discover the lair was pounced on by everyone with nerve-wracking shrieks. He or she was then declared demonstrable loser.

On this occasion after ten minutes' search Donald's hiding place could not be located, so we were all summoned to tea and the party proceeded without its host. Two hours later when every crumb and every jelly had been consumed and we were all leaving, a dishevelled dirt-stained, dust-covered Donald appeared. He had been amongst the rafters of a quite inaccessible attic and had missed his whole birthday party. Tears were not very far away.

In those years I was in turn enamoured of all the girls but never achieved anything more intimate than the holding of a limp hand in the Victory cinema, Loughborough or bestowing a tight-lipped kiss when on a front doorstep. My lack of enterprise in this field was due to my mother, who I'm sure succeeded in retarding my sexual development by several years. This was achieved by solemn warnings of perpetual disgrace if I committed any of the four deadly sins of such activities. These were, getting someone in the family way, being sued for breach of promise, being cited as a co-respondent, and contracting V.D. Apart from the first, which had a natural and in the circumstances happy default much later, I have so far avoided the others.

This philosophy was perhaps a factor in my turning to the fantasy world of the glittering stars on the silver screen. I went to the cinema twice and sometimes three times a week in both Leicester and Loughborough. I subscribed to every number of *Picturegoer* and *Film World* and could recite with actions sections of dialogue from *Grand Hotel, Dr. Jekyll and Mr. Hyde,* and *The Mummy.* Boris Karloff held a grim and terrifying attraction for me and when, many years later, I was to examine him in Wimpole Street I was in a way slightly disappointed to find him a distinguished looking, beautifully mannered, benevolent English gentleman.

The screen image dies hard however, and at one New Year's Eve party held by my play-agent Margery Vosper, and where Boris was a guest, her five-year-old son John, no doubt awakened by the noise of revelry, uttered piercing screams from his bedroom. Being the doctor present I went with Margery to calm him down and offer reassurance about the insubstantial nature of his nightmare which he was unable to articulate. I found the boy's mother's soothing solace highly ironic:

'Now lie down John, there's nothing to be afraid of,' she said, 'I'll ask Uncle Boris Karloff to come in and tell you a bedtime story.'

It was on holiday in North Wales that I was to discover my life-long passion for watercolour painting. We had been accompanied by a middle-aged bachelor friend of my father's from Melton, named H.B. Hewlett. Although a geologist by profession, Hewlett was also a highly accomplished watercolourist under the classical influence of David Cox and John Sell Cotman. As we were picnicking on the shore of Llyn Idwal, I became bored – at the age of eleven – of throwing stones into the placid reflections of the towering peaks and cwms and screes on the far side of the water. Gradually I wandered over to Harold and soon became absorbed by his seemingly magic transformation of a sheet of white rough stretched Whatman paper by the laying of transparent washes, into a whole picture of soft yet glowing shapes of impeccable exactitude. It was all done so quickly, and seemingly so easily that I pestered him to show me how to do it.

I was not to achieve anything like his facility for many struggling painstaking years, but the next day my father persuaded his old friend to give the little lad a lesson – one of many to follow.

Hewlett consented a trifle grudgingly. That first lesson was not at all the fun I thought it was going to be. H.B.H. was a formidable taskmaster, a veritable martinet for accuracy. He taught me to look and see and record so that I was almost in tears at the end of one hour's endeavour. But the habit of observation never left me and in medicine later it proved a valuable asset.

'We will draw those pine trees on the top of that hill,' he said.

I began with a rapid zigzag line across the paper. An India rubber slapped down beside me.

'Rub that out,' was the order. 'You're not a post-impressionist yet. I want each tree drawn to proportion from left to right, the tall ones, the short ones, the thick trunks and the thin trunks. Then we'll do the shadows. Start again.'

This time I took very very much longer. Harold surveyed my effort carefully and then sniffed. The rubber came down on the paper once more.

'You've left three trees out,' he said.

'Does it matter?' I asked astutely.

'Of course it matters,' he snorted. 'If you can't count a line of trees how do you think you'll be able to draw a whole wood?'

Some phrase on the subject seemed vaguely to come to mind.

'Besides,' he added, 'in order to learn the most difficult part of painting, which is what to leave out, you have to know what to put in, in the first place.'

I absorbed this axiom with some reservation and rubbed away at my pencil lines. The paper – I was only allowed cartridge quality – was becoming decidedly thin in places, as I slowly drew the tree tops. I began to hate the whole prospect and then found strangely that I could almost draw those trees with my eyes shut.

'That's better,' came the voice from behind me. 'Good boy. All right. Pack up. That'll do for today.'

'But what about the paints? Aren't I going to paint them?'

H.B.H. was lighting his pipe. 'In due course, boy, in due course.'

'But when?' I asked irritably.

He ruffled my hair and chuckled. 'You don't want to run before you can walk, do you?' and strode away across the springy hilly turf in his studded walking brogues and plus fours.

And so I persevered for some years, on my own, and from time to time with H.B.H. until the techniques began to come easily – perspective, the dry brush, the wet in wet. I suffered the agonies of the watercolourist; the mistake half-way through a painting which cannot be rectified as with oils, and the tearing up of the sheet; the starting again; the never knowing whether you were going to get to a satisfactory conclusion or not, until you actually got there. I learnt to cope with difficulties on site: wind, rain, clouds that altered all the tone values, flies, and patronizing spectators. As with the butterflies and moths the names of the colours, the words, increasingly charmed me – Rose Madder, Raw Sienna, Cerulean Blue, Naples Yellow and Burnt Umber. Even now I am filled with astonishment that after the inevitable period when all seems to be going wrong, fortitude and painful perseverance ultimately triumph, and there at last is a picture as one has wanted it or almost anyway.

Later, I tried oils for some time, being affected by the French condescension about the English. Watercolours were not really painting – *'les petites aquarelles, charmantes en effet, mais elles ne sont pas serieuses'*. But I came back again and again to the soft light and fleeting shadows the English climate naturally dictates and which only watercolours can capture. However, I was so stung by these Gallic criticisms that a few summers ago, being an addict of Cézanne, I took a holiday in Aix-en-Provence, to prove once and for all that a watercolour *could* capture that fierce light and those brilliant colours. Unhappily the week I went, Cézanne's permanent collection was closed *'pour réparations'* and his *Atelier* shut temporarily for unknown reasons. Nevertheless, I used to go out daily to the sites of his famous landscapes – the road to Tholonet, the Mont St.Victoire – and ply my amateur sable dipped in water with added glycerine to delay drying in the Provencal heat. The porter at the hotel observed my departures and returns with amusement. When I complained abut the closures of Cézanne's exhibition and studio, he shrugged and smiled. 'It does not matter, Monsieur. Sign your pictures "Cézanne". There are always people who will believe you.' He thought it a great joke.

The exercise was not without its reward however. I learnt two things. One was that most of the master's compositions I had envied did not arise from a genius's arrangement of spatial relationships. Wherever one looked, there they were, hundreds of perfect compositions. The trees did not have to be counted; just put down, and perhaps a few left out. The second thing was, that when I got the paintings home, at least three of the dozen or so I had executed showed that watercolours *could* capture the light and space and indigo shadows of the *Paysage Cézanne*. And moreover not all the *aquarelles* were as *petite* as all that.

It was not until 1976 that I ventured sending anything in to the Royal Academy Summer Exhibition, still to a large extent pooh-poohed by the 'real' artists. To my surprise one of the three pictures I submitted was exhibited and to my great joy was hung next to two pictures by John Nash, another of my heroes.

With some pride I attended the Varnishing Day. Formerly the exhibitors used to add finishing touches and varnish to their works after the various rooms had been settled by the hanging committees, but the occasion is now an excuse for a binge and jolly-up by the exhibitors.

As I mounted the flight of shallow marble steps with my exhibitor's ticket, I was slapped on the shoulder by a man of my age. His prominent ears and dancing eyes took me right back in time to the thirties. Kyffin Williams, now a well-established R.A. and professional teacher, had always won Mrs. Hardy's Drawing Prize awarded each year at Shrewsbury. I was always second, until he left a year before me and then I won the prize.

'How are you?' he grinned cordially. 'Got one in?'

'Yes,' I said.

'Good show, let's go and look at it.'

He stood in front of my exhibit regarding it in silence for a full minute.

'Not bad,' he said. 'But cut down the cobalt, and use French Ultramarine. Congratulations.'

A bell jangled and I then witnessed a most extraordinary scene. Tables were set out, groaning under a superb buffet: fresh salmon, cold chicken, duck, roast beef, and dozens of salads. Another table held wine glasses filled with quite a passable claret, and a very acceptable Chablis. From all corners and directions the artists descended on the feast and jostled, even bucked and bored to fill their plates. In less than five minutes the sumptuous spread had been cleared as though a swarm of locusts had swept down Piccadilly and whooshed into Burlington House to demolish it. Around the walls they sat, ladies in outmoded picture hats, shawls and wearing all manner of coloured stockings, jeans and culottes. Boots scraped the august wooden floors. The crowd was a veritable mixture of old Bloomsbury, Rock and Pop. The conversation reached a deafening pitch. Were artists still starving as they did at the turn of the century, I wondered? Judging by today's efforts, they probably were.

I left the affair, bemused and well fed but also thrilled to see my humble name displayed by an entry in the official catalogue 'Gallery V. 409 Farm Buildings. Shipton-under-Wychwood, Oxon. November 1975.'

I have only sold several pictures in my life but have given away a hundred or more. It's very gratifying to think someone may be looking at them in places all over the world. I must confess, though, what makes things sell is a mystery to me. When I married my third wife Muriel, she brought with her to Hyde Park Gardens a picture by her former husband Michael. It was an attractive abstract design in pale cream executed in string on plaster-board, but I felt it needed livening up a bit so I blocked in the enclosed shapes of the string with bright colours in Designers' Gouache. I burnished the lot with glass paper, and spattered the surface with some of Muriel's cosmetic silver eye glitter. The effect was to produce a ceramic quality. I signed the thing with suitably illegible initials and we hung it in the hall and were intrigued by questions and praise by some serious collectors at our wedding reception.

'Picked it up near the Macht,' I said with the confidence of three champagne cocktails inside me. 'It's a . . . er . . . Loewenthal.' We even had one offer, but we refused it as we don't want to lose the joke in the future. Muriel refuses to part with it.

But the accolade for my dilettante artistic efforts which I treasure most was awarded by Helen, the wife of a very old friend Ted Eveleigh, now a Lord Justice of the Court of Appeal. When, with an expansive gesture at one of her very civilized parties, I spilt a pattern of Burgundy over her new *eau-de-nil* Wilton carpet, she responded imperturbably to my abject apologies. 'Please don't worry Ronnie. Just sign it.'

6 Location Search

Examinations are not all carried out in the consulting room. For various reasons the star may request, plead or demand the medical takes place elsewhere. On occasion I have performed my act in diverse places: tiny theatre dressing rooms, behind a sand-dune, in the corridor of a train, in an aircraft, a caravan and a car.

I remember years ago going out to Pinewood to listen to Mario Zampi's heart and chest sounds while he was in the process of noisy shooting (of a song and dance picture) on one of the stages. It was impossible to get him to keep still for more than a few seconds at at time. It was like playing a fast game of medical musical chairs.

Mostly of course the venue turns out to be in a hotel suite, a hired house or flat.

The first time I saw Bette Davis was in an Elizabethan hotel not far from London. She was sitting up in a heavily draped four-poster bed, the whole room being dimly lit by dusty chandeliers and the grey English autumn daylight which found its way weakly through the leaded lights of the mullioned windows. I noticed she was dabbing her face with a piece of cotton-wool, moistened frequently from an upended bottle of lotion. I observed several pink raised lesions on her neck and face. I peered at them more closely using my pen-torch.

'Well, doctor?' she asked in her well-known amused and challenging tone. 'What's the diagnosis?'

'Bites,' I said.

'Bugs,' she nodded. 'This place is infested. I'm suing them for all they've got. I'm also leaving for the Savoy in half an hour. Unless you also want to get eaten, I suggest you do the medical later in the day. How about six o'clock and we can have a drink?'

I was dismissed but the invitation was as irresistible as her charming smile.

'Right,' I said, 'see you then.'

She went on dabbing away and I beat a retreat, wondering what camera problems were going to arise. By the time I reached one of the river suites the Savoy doctor had already changed the local application to something less heroic than her self-administered TCP and all went well with the picture. Miss Davis made a rapid recovery. I don't know whether the same could be said for the Tudor hostelry.

Examining in the frequent locale of various five-star hotel suites, as opposed to the consulting room carries the risk of interruptions and diversions which prolong the whole procedure. Telephone calls from agents, producers, the press, relatives, friends or enemies, are indeed a bugbear. During one session in the Oliver Messel Suite at the Dorchester, Elizabeth Taylor broke the flow of my clinical expertise by receiving two calls from Hollywood, made an outgoing call to New York, had a visit from a producer, and received two deliveries from the florists.

By contrast Joan Crawford at Grosvenor House was business-like in the extreme. When the phone rang she answered it with a crisp 'Miss Crawford's maid speaking . . . I'll give her the message. Thank you,' and rang off. Then to me, 'Carry on, doctor.'

I was just about to place a thermometer under Maria Callas's celebrated tongue, when she decided to use it rapidly and fortissimo by taking a phone-call. I presumed it was from Greece. In any event she spoke in rapid Greek, a language so vigorous I can never decide whether people are being merely animated or indulging in a blazing row with the person at the other end of the line. I stood with the thermometer raised in my hand as if it were the mini-baton of a paralysed conductor for what seemed like the whole length of the first act of *La Traviata*.

Errol Flynn in his private life was as flamboyant as many of his screen-roles. Having welcomed me effusively, he conducted me through three rooms of his Savoy suite, in each of which were a number of ladies, passing the time of day in a variety of ways, and in a variety of states of dress and undress, to his bedroom. This was by contrast empty, but filled with music, a large refrigerator and an even larger table bearing dozens of bottles, decanters and goblets. Eventually I got through all the formalities, but not before I had been offered innumerable drinks, a game of poker, and the free services of one of the girls in the other room.

Years later in the self-same suite I went to see Anthony Quinn whom I had already met in Rhodes. I was ushered into one of the living-rooms and with effusive apologies he said he would have to keep me waiting a little, at the same time thrusting a piece of chunky cut-glass containing Scotch-on-the-rocks into my hand. I sat down while a tailor made final adjustments to one of Mr. Quinn's suits for the film.

'The skirt doesn't hang right,' he said.

'That's OK, Mr. Quinn. Eeessy done,' said the tailor and inserted two pins.

'The sleeves are too long.'

'OK, Mr. Quinn. Eeessy done.'

'And this button is all wrong.'

'No problem.'

'What do you mean? It just doesn't damn well fit.'

'Please, Mr. Quinn. Look in the mirror.'

'Yeah, but it feels as if it doesn't fit,' Quinn growled.

'Maybe I pad the shoulders, a little, make them wider?' That did it.

'Are you telling me I haven't got natural broad shoulders . . .?' Quinn bellowed.

'No : . . er . . .'

'Yes you are.' Quinn called towards the next room. 'Honey. Come in here. Now!'

An attractive woman appeared at the door.

'Do you know what this gimp says?'

'No darling.'

'My shoulders need padding! How do you like that?' Quinn ripped off the jacket and then the shirt. 'Do you ever find anything wrong with my shoulders?'

'No darling.'

Quinn turned to me.

'Hey Doc. Is there anything wrong with my shoulders?'

'As far as I can see medically, nothing at all,' I replied though I was beginning to feel very sorry for the tailor, whose face was one of complete dismay.

'I was only suggesting . . .' he began. The jacket struck him in the chest.

'Take it away. Go back and start all over again. And be round here with it first thing tomorrow.'

'Er . . . Yes, sir,' said the tailor.

The tailor gathered up the jacket and his things and sped for the

door where he turned,
'Mr. Quinn . . .' he pleaded.
'Out!' said Quinn.
The tailor disappeared.
Anthony Quinn turned to me, an expression of sweetness and light on his features.
'OK Doc. Sorry I kept you. Some people just don't know their job.' He stripped down to his pants and thrust out his chest. I approached him with my stethoscope at the ready. He fixed me with a smile and narrowed eyes. 'So the shoulders are OK huh?'
'Magnificent,' I said.

Stanley Kubrick, an old friend through many years and who sends me a handsome gift every Christmas without fail, always insists on being examined up at his house in Elstree. This involves taking a portable X-Ray machine and doing an electro-cardiogram on site, but then Stanley is a great director who spends months on the preparation of his films in a state of continuous high mental concentration. He does not like to be disturbed during this period.

The first time I visited his eyrie, it was with some trepidation that I read the large letters painted right across the whole width of the ten foot high solid wooden gates to the courtyard:

'BEWARE OF THE DOG'

I got out of the car and went to the cast iron ring of the handle on the gate. As a precaution, I rattled it. There was no answering deep-throated roar or bark, nor the scrabbling of long-nailed paws on the other side of the wood. This encouraged me for I was expecting to hear something like the Hound of the Baskervilles.

Tentatively I opened the gate and tiptoed inside. From the building an elderly spaniel padded across the space between us. He wagged his tail and licked my hand.

Stanley is just as amiable.

Drugs, alcohol, hypochondria and temperament are factors which have to be taken into account in insurance assessment. The question about daily consumption of alcohol is always preceded by a pause and usually an underestimation. The subject is highly emotive and I know from personal experience how easy it is to make a false statement. I myself when I was about thirty went to a colleague for a life examination. We had met on many occasions with mutual dislike. I stated that I drank two bottles of claret a week. When I received notification that I was considered uninsurable I was alarmed as well as furious. I had myself thoroughly checked by another colleague and nothing amiss could be found to account for the decision. I rang my policy examiner but playing things entirely by the book he said he was unable to divulge any medical findings to a proposer even if he were a doctor. The company were equally adamant. It is a very serious matter to be turned down flat, since the information is circulated to all the other life companies.

I had two virtually sleepless nights but on the third I awoke with a start and in a sweat. I remembered that what I had in fact said was 'Two bottles of claret a day!' – a clear case of wish fulfilment. Eventually I convinced another company of my mistake and so obtained the necessary policy on a first-class basis.

The film-artiste alcoholics are usually well known to the company and allowances are made. But it was impossible to overlook the late Robert Newton's performance. He took two steps into the consulting room, cried,

'Jim, lad . . .'

and fell over.

There are those who so fear that something sinister will be found that they exhibit a tremor, a very rapid pulse, and dilated pupils. A little verbal anaesthesia and reassurance usually calm them down. Richard Harris's reactions are very different. He has a robust constitution and is one of the fittest men I have ever examined. He so dislikes medicals, however, that at one time he used to ring me some fifteen minutes or so after his appointment saying he was held up in a pub a mile away and would I like a jar and go and examine him there. This was neither a practical nor professional procedure. I said I would wait for him. After another twenty minutes he rang again.

'I'm sorry doctor, but I've been held up again . . .'

'Where are you now?' I asked. He named another pub half a mile nearer.

After one more call from a pub a few hundred yards away, he eventually arrived, absolutely sober and over one hour late. The physical findings were flawless. I suggested that he might pay my fee on a geometrical progressive basis in future related to the number of stops on the way. He readily agreed, though this was never put into practice. On conclusion of the examination we went out and had an enjoyable couple of drinks together.

Some people are so obsessive that they insist on mentioning in minute detail all the trivial medical events of their lives like ingrowing toenails and the removal of warts. Such details fill up the form to an alarming degree and run the danger of their being turned down as a result of a mere glance at the word-laden paper by the underwriter.

Others are full of delusional fears and mis-information like the girl who said she had had two brain tumours and varicose veins of the arms. This latter condition could probably only occur if she had been walking on her hands since birth.

Hypochondria is the fear of disease or the belief in imaginary illness. Most neuroses are based on fear of one thing or another. A very common one is of travelling. I have probably inherited a degree of this, now happily virtually conquered, from my parents. My father so disliked driving a car that he tried to combat this by a show of indifference to other road users, and a determination to complete a journey in the shortest possible time, and hence at the greatest possible speed. This produced two very unnerving driving habits. If he was going along an empty straight road, when an approaching vehicle appeared in the distance he would accelerate and begin admiring the countryside. Though there was ample room for the two vehicles, by the time they passed each other, he had eased the car nearer and nearer to the centre, so that when they passed there was barely a coat of cellulose between them. His second habit was that he so hated changing down, once in top gear, that he relied entirely on steering to get through a market town such as Loughborough to the consternation of other drivers, pedestrians, and police. The repetition of these experiences caused my mother, who was very religious, to put down her head and pray sometimes audibly, or perhaps guiltily sing a hymn.

I never owned a motor-cycle, and certainly now never will, not least because of memories of a pillion journey through Snowdonia behind my old friend Denys Johnson during a thunderstorm, and a free ride on Laurence Harvey's newly acquired moped round the medical area at the end of one of his examinations.

My first wife Thelma was not made for twentieth century travel: She once clocked up fourteen miles on a shopping trip from Weymouth Street to Bond Street and back – a geographical distance of three miles.

Her natural distrust of things mechanical was only confirmed by her experiences on the night train to Munich. I had to examine a member of the cast of a Michael Winner film there and it had been decided that she and the girls should accompany me on the trip. As soon as the train moved out from the station Thelma became convinced that there was something mechanically and seriously wrong with the wheels of the carriage. Repeatedly and irritably I told her nothing was amiss and that the rolling and banging were quite standard and par for the course in a *wagon-lit*. Exhausted by this exchange, but at last dozing off about 1 a.m. I came to with a deafening crash, violent braking and a precipitate fall from the upper bunk. Shouts from outside of '*Raus, Raus!*' gave the impression that we had slipped back in time to World War Two and we had arrived at our concentration camp destination.

In fact, the wheels right under us had indeed broken. With Thelma giving me triumphant looks indicating that intuition was an infallible asset, we were bundled out, half-dressed and with hastily repacked cases, hurried along a station platform and deposited in unheated couchettes. Remonstrations with the German officials that we were first-class passengers were met with quick assurances that we would be compensated. To the German mind, the most important aspect of the crash was that the coach had lost eight minutes of its time, which must be caught up as German trains were never late. Needless to say we arrived in Munich absolutely on time.

Having deposited the family at the *Vierjahrzeiten*, I was still sore and tetchy by noon when I had a consultation with a Munich physician over an artiste he had turned down for insurance. The basis for this rejection was a listing of three fainting attacks. Further investigations would be necessary. This would involve time and a recast of her part, much to her extreme disappointment.

The lady in question was in her late twenties, had twice been a skiing champion and was in magnificent shape, if not a veritable Brünnhilde. A few questions disclosed that each attack of the vapours had occurred on leaping up from bed on the first day of her menses.

Our medical discussion was conducted through the medium of an interpreter and when I pointed out that I considered the attacks were physiological not pathological, and in my opinion the artiste was perfectly fit to act in the film, my Teutonic colleague leapt to his feet and harangued me in his own inimitable language. I gathered that he considered it an insult that a '*verdampt Englander*' should question his opinion. I asked the interpreter to ask him to calm and also sit down or I would be obliged to stand up too. The artiste was by now in tears and all four of us stood while the tirade continued. At last it ceased, a smile appeared on the other doctor's features, he thrust out his hand and shook mine. I left shortly afterwards and invited him for a drink that evening at the hotel and to meet my family. He clicked his heels and nodded, but never showed up. The artiste made a very successful debut in her first English-speaking picture.

I imagine most people have in greater or lesser degree a healthy fear of flying. When alone I frequently seem to be seated next to a Scottish engineer (it must be the same man in different disguises) who regales me with stories of hazardous flights and the multiple small mechanical faults in an aircraft which can spell disaster. I am sure as a result of his influence I noticed on a flight to Amman on one of the early Comets, that one of the eight bolts holding the window beside me was frosted with ice. I don't think I would have been too worried if the other seven had been the same; but the odd man out bugged me.

It meant that at best the other seven were at fault. Eventually I plucked up enough courage to ask the co-pilot on his tour of the passengers' cabin if the anomaly of the single frosted bolt had any dangerous significance. He examined the offending object and then treated me to a thin smile.

'At this altitude,' he said, 'such a thing is quite standard.'

'But why one . . .?'

'You're perfectly safe, sir,' he cut in pityingly and moved on down the gangway.

The Scottish engineer at my side squinted and shook his head sadly. Reassuringly he put his hand on my arm.

'There's nothing you can do, laddie,' he said. 'Except pray.'

The fear of looking a frightened fool is so strong, stronger than logic or the contemplation of catastrophe that I sat in silence until we touched down safely.

But the spirit of self-preservation dies hard and a few years later I refused to board a plane at Hamburg for West Berlin, because as I approached the steps up to the cabin I had to walk across at least thirty yards of tarmac soaked in kerosene. The German airport personnel were furious and explained the leak was not from the aircraft but an overflow from the servicing bowser. I was not convinced, much to the embarrassment of Jim Guild of E.I.A. and Robin Hillyard of Ruben Sedgwick who were accompanying me to the medical I was to perform on a director of a film, who was developing neurotic symptoms and erratic behaviour. I returned, in spite of entreaties, to the lounge for a coffee. After ten minutes the pilot appeared and conducted me across the tarmac. The kerosene had been dispersed with German efficiency and once more feeling very foolish I climbed up into the plane which took off faultlessly.

After that, I don't think now I would make any comment if a wing of a Boeing dropped off in flight.

Finally in this sort of context I should mention the case of Percy Herbert. Very many of us suffer from a fear of flying. In Percy's case this is of an extreme degree. He and John Cuthbertson and I had to fly together from Athens to Rhodes for the *Guns of Navarone*. At the airport I dispensed some Sodium Amytal to help Percy on the trip – I may say to little avail. When we sat in the plane waiting for take-off, Percy clutched the seat arms and kept his gaze on the floor, refusing offers of soft drinks or a magazine from the pretty hostess, the better to control himself for the ordeal ahead. As we taxied forward suddenly he looked up and asked hoarsely, 'What's that sound? What's the noise? Can't you hear it?'

'Don't worry about that,' said John Cuthbertson with obvious pleasure. 'That's just a fault in the hydraulic system!'

Percy looked as though he was going to attempt to jump off. However, he was suitably dissuaded and he remained pale, rigid and silent until we landed. The relief that the flight was over produced unbounded release for Percy, who jumped up and began shaking everyone by the hand and kissing the hostess. We restrained him, with some difficulty, from repeating the process with the pilot.

Such are the chances of life that two hours later I was asked to see Percy in his room at the location hotel. He was swathed in dozens of towels round his body, lying in bed, his limbs flapping helplessly from each end, the treatment prescribed by the local Greek doctor. Percy had strained his back playing table tennis with the production manager. I released him and he played his part, but I believe he returned home by boat and overland transport.

7 'Kill that Baby!'

The first time I visited a film studio was at Pinewood. I had hoped to make a quick examination in a dressing-room and then be on my way back to London. But shooting was in progress, and I was invited by the First Assistant to go on the stage and watch proceedings until a suitable break occurred.

There appeared to be a very large number of people standing about doing nothing in what seemed to be a cavernous dust and hessian-smelling disused aircraft hanger, but I was assured that they all had their allotted tasks. The tenth 'take' was being prepared. What intrigued me was the jargon of the film makers. High above the floor men sat on girders and beams where hundreds of lights shone down at different angles to illuminate the scene below to the requirements of the lighting cameraman and the director. Two particular calls which were bellowed out to the minions on high puzzled me: 'Make it Chinese' and 'Kill that baby'.

I learnt that the first meant rotate the slit on a floodlight from a vertical to a horizontal axis – an anatomical reference which has no basis in fact at all – and the second was merely a request to extinguish a baby spotlight.

In retrospect I have – perhaps fancifully – likened this gruesome incitement to infanticide to my own situation when I went to Shrewsbury for my first term in the autumn of 1934.

Much has been written about the atmosphere and activities carried on in the English public school, an institution which still bewilders parents and children of most other nations – from the vivid prose of Dickens, Vachel's *The Hill*, *Tom Brown's Schooldays*, F.E. Anstey's *Vice Versa* and Hilton's *Goodbye Mr. Chips* (all filmed by Americans with varying sentimentality and inaccuracy) to the widely read boys' weekly papers of the twenties and thirties, notably the *Gem* and *Magnet* where the heroes and villains of Greyfriars, Harry Wharton, Bob Cherry, and Billy Bunter, have become immortal names in the English language if not English literature. The social revolution of the last three decades, I understand, has changed these establishments to a degree. But they remain a target for fury, denigration and class hatred by the left everywhere, though I suspect these emotions hide an underlying envy, even grudging respect. The public schools are still very much alive and kicking. Certainly the waiting lists for entry to them are almost as long as those for the benefits of socialized medicine.

I think the simplest and most illuminating comment about this strange English form of education was made in World War II – or so the story has it. Two British officers, prisoners of the Japanese, were humping heavy loads of rock and wood up the Burma road in the humid heat, racked with dysentery and on a starvation diet. One turned to the other and offered some simple words of consolation, 'Well old boy, it's not as bad as the first term at Marlborough.'

My first term at Shrewsbury hit me between the eyes, took the smile off my face, and metaphorically kicked me up the bottom. The remembered mixture of hatred and affection I have for the place, and the mere act of survival ultimately produced a casual carefree calm, not to say indifference to later unpleasant circumstances. I think my bumptious though happy conceit was certainly in need of treatment. I certainly got it. Nothing can be worse than this, I decided (and very little was), hiding tearfully and shivering under the inadequate bedclothes in an icy bedroom, where the wind blew through the permanently open but barred windows from across the Welsh Marches. George Borrow in Lavengro could not have described it better:

'There's likewise a wind on the heath.'

Like all closed societies, including the Mafia, Communist Russia, the Armed Forces or Truman's Kitchen, the basic message was one of a series of clichés:

41

'You can't beat the system'; 'You can't fight City Hall!'; 'If you try they'll get you!' They undoubtedly got me.

My father's salary at the time was insufficient to meet the fees at a public school, at least one of the original seven of the charter, Eton, Harrow, Rugby, Winchester, Charterhouse, Westminster and Shrewsbury. Lesser targets were not considered. So the only way for me to meet some of the cost was to win a scholarship. I was thus crammed and coached in my weaker subjects, Latin and History, my strength lying in English, Physics, Chemistry, Geography, French and Mathematics. I was an unusual candidate because I did not share the background of my competitors. They had all been to private prep schools, not a co-educational state grammar school; the uniqueness of this fact was soon impressed upon me. Shrewsbury was my own first choice simply because I had just read the novel about the school by Desmond Coke called *The Bending of a Twig*. The sentence about the hero at the end of one chapter haunted my dreams. 'Shrewsbury was gradually weaving its spell about him.'

I still believed every word of it as I went on the train from Leicester with my mother, who stayed with me in the town for the three days of the papers and vivas ahead. I remember her testing me all the way in the carriage on the irregular Latin verbs in Kennedy's *Latin Primer* 'Tango, tangere, tetigi, tactum; Pingo, pingere, pinxi, pictum' and the rhymes to aid the memory 'Common are to either sex, artifex and opifex. Conviva, vates, advena, testis, civis, incola . . .'

On a sunlit early May morning on my way to the first test, I paused on Kingsland toll bridge, clutching my pencil-box, ruler and geometry instruments, and looked up to the school building, high above the magnificent curve of the River Severn. The spell was already woven – even if it was not quite the one I had dreamt about. The chapel-bell began to toll. And I knew it was tolling for me.

I recall little about the examinations but in my final viva conducted by the headmaster, H.H. Hardy, and two other masters, I was asked what my hobbies were. Priggishly I replied,

'I'm a lepidopterist, sir.'

One of the masters' eyes lit up.

'So am I,' he said. 'Have you got a Large Blue?'

My recollection of days with Jack Tatham rushing along the hedges with a butterfly net near Wymeswold and Quorn and on holidays on the South Downs, where Common Blues, Chalkhill Blues and Adonis Blues abounded, and my two well-thumbed chunky volumes of South's *Butterflies and Moths of the British*

Isles, came to my aid. I spotted the trap which had been set.

'Unfortunately not, sir,' I said. 'The Large Blue has been extinct for some years now.'

He smiled and then laughed. 'You'll do,' he said.

Ten days later a telegram came to say I had been awarded a scholarship. There were twelve out of an entry of nearly a hundred. It was for eighty pounds a year. If he cut down on his cigarettes, it was just about enough for Dad.

I spent the remainder of my last summer term at Humphrey Perkins in a state of supreme excitement. I took my School Certificate and obtained six credits which entitled me to exemption from matriculation and hence the necessary basic requirement for entry to a University. I had graduated from high school, so to speak, in order to go to another high school. This additional success to my scholarship floated me through the summer. Visits to Shipleys, the school outfitters in Leicester, to fulfil the list of clothes I would need for Shrewsbury read like an inventory for a long military campaign – 6 flannel shirts, 6 cotton shirts, 6 winter vests, 6 summer vests, 6 pairs of underpants, 1 dozen stiff Eton collars, 2 stiff white ordinary collars, 6 front studs, 6 back studs, 2 navy blue serge suits, 2 pairs grey flannel trousers, 1 tail coat and black trousers, 1 top hat, 1 straw hat or boater, 12 pairs of black socks, 2 pairs of grey games' socks, 3 pairs of black shoes, 2 football shirts, 2 football shorts, 2 fives vests, 2 woollen sweaters, 1 muffler, 1 overcoat, 1 raincoat, 2 pairs of black gloves (1 woollen), 1 pair of fives gloves, 2 pairs of plimsolls, 1 pair of football boots, 2 pairs of pyjamas, 2 blue ties, 1 black tie, 1 military hair brush and comb, 1 tuck box, 1 trunk with initials, 1 bible, 1 hymn book and 2 dozen cotton handkerchiefs, 2 pairs of linen sheets and pillow cases, and 1 travelling rug, 3 rough brown towels, 3 ordinary white towels.

For the summer term were added, 2 pairs of cricket flannels, 2 white shirts, 6 pairs of white socks, 1 pair of cricket boots and 1 cricket bat.

On to every piece of clothing my mother had to stitch a Cash's name-tape in red.

What the school provided were two old blankets, one lumpy mattress and one sagging iron framed truckle bed. I thought I was about to enter a gentleman's élite establishment of culture and education. All in all this was true. But at the time it seemed to me like open warfare.

Fred Harris, garage proprietor, motor-mechanic and village philosopher, an ardent angler and fishing partner of my father's, was co-opted into the role of chauffeur complete with peaked cap and a suitably polished and shining old Austin tourer to take me in style to No. 2 The Schools. He stopped outside the ugly Victorian House. As my mother kissed me goodbye, Fred glanced over the building noticing the iron bars (for safety of course) on the windows. He stroked his chin and said 'Goodbye Master Ronald. I think it'll take a bit of time before they butter your feet.' It did. Nearly two years.

There were five other new boys in the Reverend J. O. Whitfield's house. Philip Whitfield, his nephew, David Ellis and David Evans, Hector Layton and George Bruckshaw. Philip later became a decorated fighter-pilot and afterwards a schoolmaster; David Ellis became a surgeon; David Evans, his cousin, a solicitor – both hailed from Aberystwyth. George became an engineer and lady-killer, but I have no idea what happened to Hector. We stood foot-shifting in front of the house noticeboard reading out names on the allotted study list, warily testing each other's credentials. The rest of the forty odd boys would not arrive for two hours.

A maid came and told us Mrs. Whitfield had invited us to tea. We trooped after her into the drawing room on the private side of the house. We sat awkwardly and accepted the thick bread and butter and chocolate biscuits. No conversation took place.

Megan Whitfield was a small lady with owl-like spectacles. Her husband nearly always referred to her as 'Woman' and she to him as 'Man'. I do not think this implied that they enjoyed a rumbustious earthy sexual relationship. If it did, they certainly didn't smile much about it. In fact neither J O W nor his spouse smiled much at all. Something must have occurred from time to time, nevertheless, because she bore J O W three sons, all away at another public school. She was the daughter of a retired Housemaster and it was rumoured that there were two suitors for her hand in matrimony, J O W and Frankie Barnes, now the form-master of the Classical Shell. According to the story, Megan's father told the two admirers that the one that took Holy Orders first could marry his daughter. J O W was soon ordained and captured the prize, while Frankie remained a bachelor, romantically continuing to live nearby.We found it all quite hard to believe.

Suddenly the door burst open and our Housemaster strode into the room. He helped himself to two pieces of bread and butter, wolfing them down rapidly. He was six foot two and weighed over sixteen stone. He wore a dog collar and a bulging clerical-grey suit. It was easy to believe that he had been a Cambridge rowing blue. He stood astride, his back to the fire, and glared balefully at us for several minutes in silence, the while jingling coins in his trouser pockets, an activity crudely known in the house as playing pocket-billiards.

44

Eventually he gave us his message of welcome.

'So you're the New Scum?'

Six small boys' heads nodded hopefully.

'Well, all I have to say to you at this stage is that Scum is what you are – the lowest form of animal life in the place. For a year you will enjoy no privileges. You will just obey the rules and keep quiet, preferably keep out of sight. Any backsliding or disobedience will be reported to me. If I think the crime merits it, I will personally cut out your hearts with a large knife. Understand?'

A weak chorus of 'Yes, sirs' came from our side of the room.

'Right. Had enough tea? Good. Now cut along to Matron so that she can check your clothes list. House "tea" is at 6.30. Prayers are at 9.15 and lights out are at 10. Off you go.'

We stumbled towards the door.

'Come back,' he shouted.

We stopped dead and turned.

'Where are your manners? Thank Mrs. Whitfield for your tea.'

We did so and then beat a hasty retreat.

But J O W's bark was very much worse than his bite. Over the five years I was in his house I realized that his blustery manner hid a very kind heart. Unfortunately, older boys soon learnt how to puncture his carapace of ferocity and he could on occasion be reduced to an incoherent blustering wreck.

Richard Hillary, Battle of Britain fighter ace and war hero, was his chief tormentor. Hillary used to run back to the house after First Lesson at 7.30, steal J O W's copy of *The Times* and read it nonchalantly in the dining hall at breakfast. Eventually, J O W would come in breathing heavily from the exertion of the same journey from the school buildings.

'Hillary!' he gasped.

'Yes, sir?' Hillary replied continuing to read imperturbably.

'You've taken my *Times*: give it me back.'

'When I've finished it. Certainly sir.'

There followed an explosion inside J O W's throat and chest but he was beyond protest. He backed out defeated, making incoherent noises.

But Hillary was a very special case, as he later proved, and when in his final year J O W made one of his rare rounds of food enquiries he asked Hillary if there was anything wrong with his boiled egg.

'Yes,' replied Hillary. 'It's rock hard, I suspect rotten and quite inedible.'

To demonstrate his points, he took the egg and threw it the length of the hall. It struck the wall above Matron's ducking head and dislodged a piece of plaster the size of a dinner plate. This in turn loosened the support of a large picture of a former housemaster, which crashed to the floor with the unmistakable sound of breaking glass.

'You . . . you . . . unutterable vandal,' spluttered J O W. 'Your father will get a bill for all that immediately.'

Hillary pressed his attack in the same ruthless way that I imagine he dealt with several Messerschmitts. Smiling he said,

'My father's broke, sir.'

In those first days at Shrewsbury I felt I had entered a nightmare world. As I had never stayed away from home on my own for more than a few days, the pangs of home-sickness developed like a pall over the shower of customs (to me some quite incredible and barbarous) to which I had to adapt.

The physical surroundings were stark and uncomfortable. As a 'scum' you were not allowed a cushion on the study hardwood chair. 'Two-year-olds' were and 'three-year-olds' were allowed the incredible luxury of a deckchair. The spartan conditions in the bedrooms were reinforced by a compulsory cold bath or shower before first lesson at 7.30 a.m. A hot bath was allotted two nights a week. As the roster did not allow time for change of water, the new 'scum' had the pleasure of luxuriating in the dirty water of three previous bathers. This was not as unhygienic as it might seem, because we had a hot shower after any game. Football, fives, running, and different sports were mandatory at least once and often twice a day.

The programme, apart from lessons and chapel, was so packed that everything seemed to be carried out at the double. Each evening from seven to nine-fifteen were 'lock-ups'. Though not literally locked into one's study, a step outside the door was a beating offence. One was not allowed to speak, unless spoken to, to anyone who had been in the school more than one year. This apparently left a hundred contemporaries with whom one could converse, but in fact this was reduced to about five or six because friendship with any boy in any of the twelve boarding houses except one's own produced suspicion of homosexual practices.

In the study measuring six foot by eight, the new 'scum' sat at the centre desk with a 'two-year-old' by the window and the 'three-year-old' – the study monitor – by the door. During 'lock-ups' when work was supposed to be done I soon found I was the captive plaything of the other two senior boys, in my case one called Binton and one called Ruffley. Often I was shoved under my desk for the whole session, four feet pounding me at intervals.

When the bell went for tea, I emerged with my clothes covered in dust and dirt. This resulted in a dressing-down from Matron if not from the Head of House or J O W. Excuses were useless.

Binton and Ruffley certainly made my life hell. But the power and terrifying stature of these bigger, older boys diminished as I grew larger. Eventually they left long before me. I never saw Ruffley again, but one day thirty years later I recognized Binton – a strangely pathetic figure shuffling down Marylebone High Street. I went up behind him and slapped a hand on his shoulder and shouted 'Binton. Stand up straight.' He swung round with startled eyes.

'What? W . . . what?' he stammered. 'Who are you?'

I suddenly felt ashamed at frightening this grey older careworn man.

'I'm sorry,' I said. 'I mistook you for someone else.'

He smiled wanly. 'That's all right. Easily done.' He turned and continued on his way.

Rather more unpleasant forms of bullying were to be endured in silence. The brush-trick consisted of several sharp slaps on the back of the hand with the stiff bristles of a hair or clothes brush. This was followed by vigorous windmill circling of the arms until small beads of blood appeared from the microscopic puncture wounds caused by the bristles. Though I never personally suffered it, in some cases nails were knocked through the wooden seat of the chair while another boy sat heavily on one's knees.

I soon discovered that any presents from home of food, fruit, chocolates, biscuits were immediately devoured by one's study-mates. Gerry Horlick overcame this by having sent him a hundredweight of his family's celebrated malted-milk tablets. This did not prevent constant denigration of the product by praising the rival beverage Ovaltine, which used to precipitate in him an uncontrollable rage. Sadly, Gerry was killed in the Royal Navy soon after war broke out.

I managed to buy some peace from my study-mates because as a scholar I was academically way above them and found it easy to do their maths problems. No one seemed to notice that they both suddenly began scoring high marks which brought encouraging comment on their performance in the half-term and terminal reports.

The ordeal was furthered in the bedroom where the bedroom-monitor held sway. Misdemeanours were dealt with by an offer of a beating, which was a choice of three with a towel-rail, five with a slipper or twenty with the back of a tooth-brush. Certain rumoured bedroom practices were stopped eventually by the authorities. One was giving enemas with a bicycle pump, and the other was the 'jerry' game. In this the recipient was placed over the pot receptacle with his private parts inside. He was then shoved under a bed, and the rest of the bedroom jumped on top of it. I am glad to say that all these barbarous practices were in fact isolated cases and bullying was by no means widespread through-out the school. Character building by such methods completely stopped after World War Two.

That universal experience taught its own sickening lessons.

Outside the house other humiliations awaited me. I was assigned to Mr. Tombling's form, the Modern Shell. As a scholar I was allotted a desk on the first row in front of the master's desk. The door to the form room was at the back. It opened to admit my form-master, a tubby man with a beetling brow and horn-rimmed spectacles. His voice was loud and menacing. When he came in I sprang to my feet and looked to the front as I had been taught at Humphrey Perkins as a courtesy to the master. I was aware of sniggers behind me. Half-turning I noticed that no one else was standing up. I began to blush but to sit down would be an ignominious admission that I had done the wrong thing, done what was 'not done'. A streak of stubbornness made me remain on my feet. Tombling puffed his way to the front of the form and mounted the master's dais, banged a pile of new textbooks on his desk, polished his glasses and then hitched up his gown. The two of us stood exchanging a long eyeball to eyeball stare. Suddenly he bellowed at me.

'What's the matter with you, boy? Siddown!'

I obeyed with alacrity and the sniggers became outright laughter. Tombling held up his hand. The laughter died away. He stepped off the dais and started to distribute the textbooks, *Caesar's Gallic War – Book one.* When he gave me mine, he asked,

'What's your name?'

'Thorn, sir.'

'Oh yes. I've heard about you. Got your School Certificate already I understand. Well, you're going to have to take it all again in two years' time. Scholar aren't you? Strong in maths and science? Well let's hear you construe a bit of Caesar. Start at page one. Read it out.' I opened the book and began the famous first sentence.

' "*Gallia in tres partes divisa est . . .*" '

'Stand up boy when you "stru",' he shouted.

I did so. And my first lesson at Shrewsbury proceeded for me in total misery. Because of my weakness in Latin I came nearly bottom at the end of the first term, but by the end of the third I had crept my way up to the top. As my confidence returned during that year I still never forgave Tombling for that initial humiliating experience. I detemined to get my own back, and managed it with the assistance of an overweight boy called Rudder. He had distinguished himself by eating eighteen hard-boiled eggs in the school shop as a wager. The feat was performed in front of a large crowd, before he collapsed on the floor in a groaning twitching state. I think this gave me the idea. Tombling was in the habit of dealing a blow with a book behind the ears to any boy who made a mistake in Latin translation. Rudder, who frequently collected cranial blows, was persuaded to have a fit. I had supplied him with a small paper bag of Eno's Fruit Salts to hold in his mouth.

In due course Tombling delivered his attack. Rudder conducted a very creditable performance. He leapt up with a cry, began shaking and jactitating and then flung himself to the floor and bit into his Eno's bag, producing a large foaming mass from his mouth while rolling his eyes.

By pre-arrangement the whole form rose to its feet and pandemonium broke loose. Windows were thrust up and down, desk lids banged and the door opened and closed repeatedly. Cries from all sides assailed the astonished Tombling, his face blanching.

'You've killed him, sir.'

'He's definitely unconscious, sir.'

'Shall I fetch a doctor?'

'Shall I get the headmaster, sir?' and so on.

Tombling personally helped Rudder to his feet.

'Two of you . . . take him back to his house. And everybody sit down.'

Rudder, myself and another boy departed obediently. As far as I know Tombling never used a book as a weapon again.

I found the fagging system (or 'Daouling' as it was called after the Greek Doulos, a slave) utterly preposterous. A monitor would call 'Daoul'. All new 'scum' had to drop everything and run to the monitor. The last to arrive got the job. This could entail running an errand, cleaning football boots or going to the semi-exterior 'Lats' and warming the lavatory seat with one's bottom until the monitor arrived to perform his defecation.

I was overcome by a sense of bewilderment and a feeling of helpless imprisonment. There was no one to whom to appeal. Any complaints were met with chastisement. At least six times a day the roll-call was taken, in the house, in the chapel, at every lesson and at prayers in the evening. It seemed to me that escape, which was very much in my mind, was about as difficult as a break from Alcatraz. There was a 'window', however, of about two hours in the afternoon on a Wednesday half holiday when I felt it could be achieved. I got as far as the railway station at my first attempt. But the ticket-office personnel were used to the game and refused to sell me a ticket. A phone-call to the school brought the Head of

House down in twenty minutes, and I was conducted back in silence.

My second attempt in which I managed to ring my mother from a coin-box failed because my incoherent pleas for her to come and fetch me, were followed by my father's voice on the line telling me calmly to go back to school and that he and my mother would come at the weekend and see Mr. Whitfield.

Before they arrived, however, in the two days which had to elapse an additional stress had been added to my near-breaking spirit.

As a result of a defect in development of the cartilaginous plates on each side of the bodies of the vertebrae I had a 'roundback' – Schauermann's syndrome. This deformity was noted by the boys, Matron and Mr. Whitfield who for years used to put his knee in my back as I stood washing at the basin in the bedroom.

'Stand up Thorn. Put your shoulders back.'

One day when I was much older I told him,

'Sir, it's quite pointless doing and saying that. It is an anatomical deformity. I find it also repetitive and boring, so kindly don't do it again.'

He looked hurt and turned away. But he didn't repeat the procedure. My protest also earned me a new respect from my bedfellows.

Long before this though, in the first two weeks which nearly broke me down, I was handed over to the equal medical ignorance of Sergeant Major Joyce who ran the gymnasium. He was given when urging us over the 'horse' to shout 'Guts and grind yer teeth. Fight for the British Empire!' He proclaimed that my trouble was 'all dorsal, all dorsal' and instituted a procedure to straighten my back. I had to hang from a high bar on the wallbars, my back to them, while another boy climbed up under me until I was arched outwards, my feet dangling. Sergeant Major Joyce then grasped my ankles and forced them back towards the wall. The pain was formidable. At the second treatment I felt an agonizing wrench in my left hip. He had succeeded in slipping the epiphysis of the head of my left femur. I crashed to the floor in a fainting state. The pain subsided to a large degree but Joyce was obviously disturbed as I scrambled away. The incident was referred to the school doctor who visited each house about three times a week. Observing my limp and miserable demeanour he gave my leg a perfunctory examination and declared his diagnosis.

'Malingering, Matron. He can play full games.'

And that is what I did. The trouble settled down except for intermittent aching. In due course I scored goals in house matches and was in the fourth eleven at cricket and went to camp with the O.T.C. I played golf, tennis and squash until I was forty but the gradual development of a severe arthritic hip led to a disability in my late fifties. I was completely delivered from this by a total hip replacement in 1981 carried out by John Strachan and my old friend Professor Lipmann-Kessel. The hip is totally pain-free and over ninety per cent mobile. I can do most things I haven't enjoyed for twenty years.

At the end of my first two weeks my parents came down. J O W put them in his drawing room and I was summoned to join them. He left us alone. I think it was the sight of my beautiful mother which cracked me. I at last burst into tears.

They stayed the night at the Lion Hotel on Wyle Cop in Shrewsbury, and I was allowed out to spend the day with them. The sudden remembered comforts of civilized life and the feeling of kindness from loved ones seemed like an escape from the Inferno. I wanted to leave Shrewsbury and go home. But wisely my father, with reluctant agreement from my mother, put a compromise to me.

'Stick the term out, Ronald, and then we'll review the situation at Christmas.'

I went back and did just that. I'm very glad I did. Over five years those black early days were quite soon overcome, but never forgotten.

But I must confess that my resolution wavered. I arrived home for the Christmas holidays with broken chilblains on every finger and toe, and had a moment of panic. Could I face it all again? I invented my own compromise. Two days before I was due to return I went down to the potting shed at the bottom of the garden armed with a full pepper pot. I shook pepper down my throat and coughed and spluttered hard for some ten minutes. I then went back and told my mother I didn't feel well. I was gratified to discover I already had a temperature. I was put to bed.

When Dr. Gray came to see me about two hours later he inspected my throat, which was by then very sore indeed. He made a quite correct diagnosis of acute pharyngitis. He was not to know that it was traumatic and not infective.

Mr. Whitfield was rung and I returned to school a week late for the spring term. Shrewsbury continued to weave its spell. J O W had the final word. On fourteen of the fifteen terms I was there, the housemaster's comment on my end of term report was 'He is a good boy in the House.' On the last and fifteenth it changed to 'He's a good boy in the House and I like him.'

8 'Voices Over'

Most people know the apocryphal chestnut about the surgeon who is introduced by his hostess to a lady guest at a party.

'Mr. Evans, I don't think you've met Mrs. Jones.'

'No I haven't. How do you . . .?'

'Oh, but we *have* met,' interrupts Mrs. Jones. 'You operated on me last year.'

'I do apologize,' replies the surgeon blandly, 'I didn't recognize you with your clothes on.'

The converse situation can apply. At a party or other affair, in a restaurant or hotel, there have been occasions where a film artiste I have examined, has looked through, over or round me with, I am sure, genuine lack of recognition. I always make it a matter of professional etiquette to offer no facial expression in return.

I imagine these well-known personalities are so preoccupied with their own image and reputation that the world of other people outside show-business consists of a sea of nameless faces, (but all hopefully belonging to fans). The stars of course respond readily to any approach for an autograph, though they sometimes complain in private of the tedium of this activity. They are always on show and I sympathize with their occasional outbursts of irritation at finding it difficult to pursue a private life. When Garbo said she wanted to be alone she meant just that. Failure to remember me, an unknown insurance doctor, however detailed the repeated medical examinations, is very understandable.

But some doctors are human and all are subject to weaknesses. I must confess to a personal satisfaction when chance meetings have been acknowledged with charm, enthusiasm and even hospitality. I remember the look of astonishment on my first wife's and two friends' faces when we were having dinner at the old Caprice, and Yvonne de Carlo came over from her table. She embraced me effusively and showered me with questions about my welfare. She even got my name right. But then she is not only a beautiful, but a very bright lady.

While on holiday with my family at the Cap Estel on the Riviera, John Mills, and his wife Mary and daughter Hayley were also staying there. When we came down to the terrace on our first night, he immediately greeted me.

'Dr. Thorn, I presume,' he said. 'Come and join us for a drink.'

He has that enviable capacity for friendliness which is in no small part responsible for his immense popularity.

Patrick MacNee at the height of the TV Avengers series found us, again *en famille*, at a hotel at Goodwood, where we stayed one Christmas. He took off his celebrated bowler, threw his umbrella with uncanny accuracy into the stand in the hallway and beamed his way up to us.

'Hello doctor,' he said. 'What are you doing here?'

'Fleeing from the seasonal household chores and cooking,' I replied.

'What a sensible thing to do . . .' he smiled.

'A drink?' I asked.

'But of course,' he said. 'Thank you. Plenty of time before lunch.'

And we all trooped into the bar together.

Harry Andrews, when we were visiting my daughter Amanda, then in her first term at Newnham, and I was entertaining her latest boyfriend to lunch at the Garden Hotel, Cambridge, came over to our table. He reversed our roles neatly and enquired about my health. Whatever else it did, it impressed Amanda's boyfriend no end. Her reputation positively rocketed. When a little later in the term, after I had told Michael Winner at a medical before he was to make a film on location in Cambridge, that my daughter was at Newnham, without announcing his intention to me, Michael had her telephoned by the production secretary, invited her to the location, sent a car for her and gave her lunch. Such spontaneous hospitality is a rare thing indeed. Amanda thereafter worked her way through other boyfriends at alarming speed. But not just because of that.

The glitter of the stars and personalities of the entertainment world is often cast aside, I suspect with relief, at medicals. A doctor, like a priest, hears confidences the secrecy of which is sacrosanct. My card index of notes with confidential information is kept well guarded and locked away safely. I have only had one nasty moment. When I went to see Ava Gardner in her large flat in Ennismore Gardens I inadvertently dropped her card on the steps to the house as I left. By the time I reached home her maid telephoned me to say she had found the card. I rushed round immediately and retrieved it, and ascertained that no one but the maid had seen it. I rang Miss Gardner with apologies which she accepted readily, as well as the two dozen roses.

Many of the artistes find a medical examination an opportunity to relax and be themselves, and talk about matters quite outside their usual intensely enclosed world. I have had discussions about a wide variety of subjects, and have discovered a surprising interest in my life and activities. This exchange has in some cases blossomed into a ready acquaintanceship and even friendship.

Comments on the contents of my consulting room which contains some interesting things are in many instances the jumping-off point. American women are usually surprised by the decor, furniture, pictures and books which reflect my personal baroque taste. They glance round and exclaim,

'But this isn't like a doctor's office at all!'

'Do you like it?'

'I just love it. It's so . . . so . . .'

'Homey?'

'No. I guess cute would be a better word. What a very beautiful desk!'

'I spend a great deal of time at it.'

They then turn their scrutiny on to me.

'And you don't look like the usual doctor. You don't have a white coat.'

'Buttoned up to the neck? With short sleeves?'

'That's right.'

'No. I'm always afraid I might be mistaken for a hairdresser.'

I have one huge oil painting by John Johnstone whose work appears in a number of national galleries – mostly South American which is odd for a Scotsman. It is a puzzle picture with reflecting mirrors and surfaces. It also has a small elephant in the corner. It is pretentiously called 'Remembrance to a Dark Afternoon'. I bought it from a gallery in Cork Street when I was a little drunk. The dominant colours are light red and turquoise – which I felt would go with the furnishings in our flat at the time. Also my wife Thelma collected ornamental elephants. It seemed I couldn't lose. But she didn't care for it, and so I put it in my consulting room. I asked my old friend Neville Main, a professional artist, what he thought of the painting. He regarded the picture for a minute or so, and then with his familiar impish grin, gave his verdict. 'Well, I will say this for it, Ronnie. It's a big 'un.'

I have grown to be fond of the thing and I find it excellent for keeping young children quiet by asking them to look at it carefully and then tell me all the things they can see in it.

On the other walls are watercolours executed by the doctor, sticking to the rules imbued by H.B. Hewlett. These have brought compliments from those actors who paint or collect pictures themselves, the most enthusiastic being from John Standing who is no slouch as an exponent himself and also from Dustin Hoffman, an ardent collector. There has been no comment about the *aquarelles* from French artistes. But then as Mandy Rice-Davies might have said, 'There wouldn't be, would there?'

The attractive Veronica Carlson paints a lot. She asked me if I'd like to see her work at her studio. I somehow never managed to get there. Maybe it was because of a male trepidation about women's lib, the female version of an invitation to look at some etchings.

I have two ornate high-backed chairs which are very comfortable. They are bogus thrones which I picked up for a song in the sale of furniture when Denham Studios closed down. There is another decorative piece, in painted wood, a copy of a priceless marble credenza in the Uffizi in Florence. I have resisted several substantial offers for it from American producers and directors. My second wife Halina dubbed it 'the Monstrosity', but Muriel adores it and so it has been moved back to our hall in Hyde Park Gardens.

Those that have come many times always notice changes, additions and subtractions.

Michael Caine is a man of sharp intelligence and an acute observer. When he last came, he had no sooner sat down in the usual patient's chair than he scanned the chimney-piece where I had some new framed photographs. No mean connoisseur of female form and beauty he pointed to a picture of Muriel.

'Who's the new bird?' he enquired.

'She's not a new bird, she's my new wife,' I told him.

'Congratulations,' he said.

Katharine Hepburn, one of the greatest and most sensitive actresses on stage or screen, perceptively observed at one examination:

'You look depressed, Dr. Thorn.'

'I am,' I replied. 'I've just had a hernia operation which went wrong and had to be repeated, and my wife left me shortly afterwards.'

'Oh God, I'm sorry,' she said, and then fixing me with a sympathetic but penetrating stare, added, 'Whose fault?'

'Neither,' I replied. 'But it has been a bit of a shock after twenty-five years.'

Miss Hepburn then gave one of her celebrated rushing anguished speeches full of genuine feeling and sensitivity.

'Doctor, I just don't understand these things . . . women can be so cruel, they really can . . . men are so vulnerable, they really are . . . I just don't understand, I really don't . . . It's so awful the things people do to each other . . . but don't let it get you down, honey . . . really don't . . .'

She put a hand on my arm briefly and smiled at me.

'You'll rise above this. You really will. Hell, you're still young.

55

How old are you?'

'Fifty-two,' I said.

She laughed.

'You've nothing to worry about. You've everything to live for. Really you have, really. You're going to be so happy in the future. I know you are. I just know it, I just feel it.'

'Thank you,' I said.

She sniffed and blew her nose and then, smiling, said:

'Don't you think we ought to get on with the physical?'

'Of course. I'm sorry,' I said.

I picked up my stethoscope, and listened to her heart. It was beating robustly and regularly. The sound gave me a message of strength and courage. Her words had begun to lift my depression. I shall always be grateful for her genuine concern and sympathy at that time.

Much later, when I told Lord Olivier I had found someone I wanted to marry, he looked at me levelly, and then said quietly, 'Yes, yes. But don't rush it. Don't for heaven's sake rush it. Say to her for a long time, "I adore you, darling. I will do anything for you darling. I will buy you everything I can down to my last penny. I will love you, darling, morning, noon and night." But don't mention the little gold band, not for a long time.'

I followed his advice except being a less experienced man, I had not the patience to obey his last injunction. I must say I have not for a second regretted this deviation.

Certain artistes I have seen so many times that I regard them as more than acquaintances. Kenny More used to call me 'The Actor's Friend'. Sir John Gielgud I regard as the intellectual of the handful of very great actors and his examinations invariably include riveting philosophical observations on behaviour and life in general, rather in the manner of his performance in *Brideshead Revisited* as Ryder's father. Each time he comes now I think of our meeting as Gielgud Revisited.

Peter Bowles is making more and more films and TV series so that I am now seeing him quite a lot. Once he arrived in an excited state. It was the day he had acquired his first Rolls-Royce. His pulse rate was definitely raised. He is a car addict and he had parked the new car on the yellow line opposite my rooms in Harley Street. The examination was conducted in fits and starts as we kept going to the window to admire and eulogize about his purchase. The last time he told me, sadly, that he had sold the Rolls as it was unsuitable for his dog, which spoilt the interior 'hair and scratchwise'. The animal is now confined more effectively in the back of his new Porsche.

Examinations of Kenneth Williams are usually prolonged because he is an indefatigable raconteur. Andrew Keir is a serious expert on the details of manufacture and variety of malt whisky. Brian Blessed brings with him such a mixture of good humour and robust health that after he has gone I feel as if I have had an intravenous injection of Parenterovite. Ray Milland, a last patient of the day, stayed for canapés and drinks. Ginger Rogers tried to convert me to vegetarianism. Leonard Rossiter admitted using one of my stories about Noel Coward in an after-dinner speech which went down very well. He did, however, quite correctly acknow-ledge the source of the anecdote. Lee Marvin is a delightfully amiable man and didn't frighten me at all.

Certain artistes I have encountered in pairs. I went to examine Lauren Bacall at the Savoy, and in the middle of the proceedings, Bogey arrived in a raincoat, hat-brim turned up, and a camera slung around his neck. He had been out photographing London, and was presumably playing an unscripted part as a tourist. He gave me a pleasant greeting with the celebrated toothy smile.

'Hello, honey,' he said to Lauren, changing his role to Philip Marlowe. 'Do you want me to take a shot of you with this guy?'

James Mason will discourse on a wide range of subjects with great knowledge. He has been known to become so engrossed that the medical examination becomes a secondary affair. I was trying to get him to concentrate on the procedure of taking his blood pressure. He rolled up a sleeve and continued talking. His wife prompted him gently,

'The other sleeve, James, the other sleeve.'

Politics sometimes raises its ugly head and I felt decidedly limp on the day that I examined Jane Fonda in the morning and Vanessa Redgrave in the afternoon. I later went out and voted for Margaret Thatcher.

In the group of long-standing personal friends is Leslie Phillips. When he was very young he played the small part of a shy policeman in a play of mine which eventually reached the West End. He stole all the notices and has been doing this ever since in countless comedy stage successes and films. Like most comedians the superbly-timed comic throwaways and subtle 'business' – he has, unkindly I think, once been dubbed King Leer – hides a serious sensitive character and a dedicated professional.

John Horsley, who is now never out of work on TV, and his wife June came to live in a flat above us when we lived in Weymouth Street. At one time his two charming daughters Sarah and Emma joined our two, Amanda and Vanessa, in daily excursions to the tennis courts in Regent's Park. Thelma and June got on well and on Sundays John and I joined them for picnics.

When I was suffering from a transient eye condition, John, who happened to be 'resting', kindly drove me all over Greater London on my visits to doctors and hospitals in connection with my medico-legal practice. The arrangement worked on the whole very well but sometimes played havoc with my itinerary, because after I had seen a patient I often returned to the outpatients hall to wait while John signed autographs for countless fans of his amongst the halt and the lame.

At times in my life when stress and calamity have overtaken me, I have received friendship, advice and sympathy from John and June, visiting them at awkward times – and often unannounced – at their house in Hendon. John has described me as a foul-weather friend.

Diane Hart, a star in her day of Shaftesbury Avenue and Broadway and in films, I have known since she played the lead in another comedy of mine. She was a great success, but I fear the play wasn't. It did sixteen weeks on a pre-London tour and then bankrupted the management, and we never came in.

More recently I came across her again when I was crawling about following my hip-replacement operation. Marigold Mann had wonderfully restored all my movements with some tough intensive physiotherapy. But I still lacked confidence. Diane with her boundless energy and drive restored that in no time at all.

As I hesitated on the pavement before crossing the road she would shout from the other side,

'Come on Ronnie, run. Sod the cars! Of course you can do it. Now, darling now!'

It certainly got me across and her professionally trained voice and authoritative gestures certainly stopped the traffic.

Bryan Forbes, who is as good a writer of books as he is a director of films, shares common ground with me as a writer as well as having a similar sense of humour. This has cemented a friendship which began years ago. There is so much to talk about when he comes to a medical, things tend to get mixed up, and I am often not sure who is examining whom. His beautiful and intelligent wife Nanette Newman often accompanies him and then the examination can develop into a medical-histrionic threesome. When I last saw them Nanette told me she had been having hypnotism to cure her of an addiction to peanuts, and had I any other ideas?

'Try prunes,' I said, but I don't know if she has taken the advice.

Because of my long period of carrying out examinations, Bryan once suggested I should have a credit on the pictures. 'Insurance Medicals by Ronald Scott Thorn', but so far, no one has taken this up.

Bryan always gives me a copy of his novels as they come out. His messages to me on the title page are always succinct and to the point. His last book which reached the top of the Best Seller list was *The Rewrite Man*. He gave me a copy, just before going off to Chicago to direct a film called *The Naked Face*. The inscription read 'To Ronnie who has seen my naked face, and a great deal else besides!'

9 Black Out

Remembrance of things past does not follow a Proustian mould for everyone. Looking back poses repeated questions. When were the first occasions of obsessive interest which became the main themes of my life? Who were the people who influenced most my thoughts and feelings? What were the shocks from which I never recovered? Why did I often fail to recognize these things at the time? Hindsight is an easy exercise. Foresight is an inspiration.

A recurrent preoccupation has always been to ponder the convoluted paths of persons who eventually cross one's own, sometimes to remain entwined for years and then to diverge or run parallel to the end. The chance encounter is remote and fascinating. The jigsaw is never completed. Pieces are mislaid or forever lost.

Great historical moments impinge on all of us. When Neville Chamberlain told us over the radio we were at war with Germany on 3 September 1939, I was sitting with my parents in the study in the school house at Barrow, towards the end of the summer holiday. At the very same moment a Polish girl named Halina of precisely my age was throwing stones at the British Embassy in Warsaw as a protest against Britain's dilatory declaration. It is amazing to think that these two events could have been connected. But over thirty years later the girl become woman and the man that was me got married. It turned out to be a mistake. The difference of nationality, experience, custom, background, religion and language proved too strong for both of us. And so we parted after six years. Perhaps I should have been warned by a painted daub on a canal bridge near my home which lasted long after the war was over. It read, 'No war for the Poles.'

When Chamberlain finished speaking, my father said something to me which has stuck in my memory. It seemed trivial at the time and quite irrelevant, but now I know it wasn't.

I was wearing a double-breasted chalk-striped grey suit, the first I had had which was not the dark-blue serge, boringly endured during the previous five years at Shrewsbury. The colour and cloth were the expression of freedom, a symbol of the new life which was to be Oxford in October, where I had gained a closed scholarship to Merton College, to read Honours Physiology and later Medicine. I was excited by the break from schoolboy conformity, symbolized by a pair of suede shoes, known amongst my contemporaries as brothel-creepers.

'You can take off those Ronald. You won't be needing them for many a year,' my father said.

'But I don't see –' I began.

'You will my boy,' he cut in. 'What is about to happen should also discourage you from giving your recent imitation of a lounge-lizard. Go and change, get outside and start filling some sandbags.'

My mother's anxious comment was,

'He'll be in a Reserved Occupation won't he, Tom?'

I went outside and did as my father asked, then helped my mother to hang the blackout curtains. The peaceful summer evening in which the late swifts darted about, and the lengthened shadows of the row of poplar trees had a magical unreality. I watched some Noctuae dart along the flower beds. It would have been a good night for 'sugaring'. It was also a good night for Panzers fanning out across the flat northern plains of Poland. But the war seemed so very, very distant. This view was strengthened next day when my uncle Morris Fox paid us a visit and gave a convincing reassurance about German air raids. 'Just wait till our anti-aircraft get at 'em.' My old friends Tom Squires and Wilf Ball arrived to build an air-raid shelter thirty yards from the house. As they sank their shovels into the rich turf and midland clay, Tom Squires said to me,

'I don't know what your father wants this dug for, they'll never get inland as far as this. Right Wilf?'

'Right Tom,' said Wilf.

When eventually we went to use the shelter for the first time over a year later, we found it under two feet of water. So instead we used the cellar in the house, the ceiling propped up with apple-tree trunks. The nearest H.E. dropped a mile away but one night we had thirty incendiaries which landed harmlessly in the orchard. At least I had a chance to use a stirrup-pump.

In my last three happy years at Shrewsbury, we were not disinterested in or cut off from the events in Spain and Europe. I remember a growing feeling of unease and gradual conviction that war was to come. Our sources of information were the Sunday press, the *London Illustrated News*, the radio and *Picture Post*. But more emphatic were the reminiscences of masters who had served in World War I, and the stories Hillary brought back after summer holidays, which he had spent alone wandering about Germany, perfecting his mastery of the language.

One master, Mr. McEachran, opened for me the whole world of poetry. Auden, Isherwood, MacNeice and Spender became a part of existence. Virginia Woolf, Hemingway and Huxley, all so totally different, were a staple diet. Even Mary Webb, sponsored by Stanley Baldwin (in addition to his growing thoughts on the aroma of Presbyterian Mixture pipe-tobacco), was read in her entirety. When the ex-Prime Minister came to give away the school prizes, the main thing I remember about him was the very limp handshake, as he presented me with my chosen book – limp probably because he may never have read a word of *The Collected Poems* of T. S. Eliot.

Personalities among the masters had their lasting effects. F.L. McCarthy really made the intricacies of biology a delight by his clear simplicity of exposition. Every living thing ultimately seemed to consist of 'a tube within a tube', and his method for marginal notes in textbooks in a graded system of sub-headings, I found unsurpassable for my later more complicated studies. Huge tomes became possible to reduce to notes on a postcard. A sheaf of these easily carried about, propped against the mirror while shaving, held in the hand during a Beethoven concert, glanced at while waiting in the pavilion before going out to bat, provided an updating of facts, a pocket memory for instant recall, the forerunner of an embryo computer. Examinations began to lose their terror. One just mentally recalled a particular postcard, and wrote out the answer.

On the lighter side, the training contrasted with that of another younger master called 'Batty' Moore who was capable of coming into the formroom and writing on the board 'Utter Gloom'. He then spent the rest of the lesson with his head buried in his folded arms over the desk. Dickie Sale's history classes were uninspiring. 'King Blank fought the battle of Blank in the year Blank. Fill in the Blanks'. Mr Pearson's maths lessons were formidable. 'And now the Binomial theorem. Binomial because it has two terms. And because it takes two terms to learn it.' Pearcrack used to take some of us out on Sundays into the country in his open tourer, a feature of which he repeatedly pointed out was 'smaller wheels – greater acceleration'. We had to do everything at the double and actually run up the nearby Shropshire hills like the Wrekin and the Breidens. On one of these a cairn of stones could be seen for miles around. Each stone had been placed on it by every boy he had taken there. We were always rewarded for these exhausting efforts by teas at a farmhouse. For four boys there were five loaves but instead of two fishes, two pounds of butter, four pounds of strawberry jam, eight pints of milk, and a dozen hard-boiled eggs.

Because of the emphasis on games and feats of the body, at which I exhibited only moderate skill, popularity seemed geared exclusively to these activities. I decided I would have to develop different if not eccentric traits. I became a very good mimic of personalities on the school site.

At Humphrey Perkins I had helped my father in the stage productions of the Old Students' Amateur Dramatic Society and had even been entrusted with the whole stage management of *The Ghost Train*. (Arnold Ridley, the author, came for an examination years and years later.) I performed in the Bump Supper entertainments and the more lavish affairs of school plays and the stage show for the Shrewsbury School Mission visit at Whitsuntide. I wrote some verse for several editions of the school magazine, and played the trumpet at every opportunity. Secretly I went to see films in the town. I remember dimly Jack and Claude Hulbert in *The Camels are Coming* and *Bulldog Jack*.

I led a food strike in the house, abetted by John Rhys who introduced mustard in a tube and cup-cakes to J O W.

I constantly changed my ambitions. Variously I wanted to be a doctor, a writer, a band-leader, an actor, an artist, a film director, a research scientist and a couturier. It is a matter of luck that I became more than one of these. My mother's desire for me to be a parson was crossed off the list very early on; no doubt the experience of Canon Blakeney played a part in this.

Gradually I made friends with other boys, breaking the rule of association outside my own house with impunity. My contemporaries, John Sharp, Richard Todd, and Peter Reynolds (Horrocks at school), all went into the acting profession and in due course came under my stethoscope – this was before the postwar days of Willie Rushton and the other old Salopian personnel of *Private Eye*. John Redway, with whom I had measles in the Sanatorium, had connections with the film world and later was my literary agent for a time. He also had Dickie Attenborough and Peter Sellers as his clients.

Thus in time I earned a certain popularity, enhanced by the visits of my glamorous mother.

Only once was my increasing prestige dimmed to the point of ostracism for some weeks following one year's school football match against Repton.

I had let it be known that my cousin Bruce Fox was the opposing team's captain. Eric Fox, my uncle, was the only really rich member of the family. Millions of Glacier mints were apparently being sucked all over the world. He not only had three cars, but a gigantic house and gardens in Leicester as well as a luxurious yacht with a permanent crew of four. He hardly ever said a word in my presence, and, at one children's tea party at his home, demonstrated his thrift and possibly the secret to his financial success, by unlocking a bureau and bringing out a tin of Fox's Glacier mints. He offered one paper-wrapped sweet to everyone present, and then solemnly locked the tin away again.

On the occasion of the Repton match he arrived with Bruce and Auntie May in a magenta and silver Rolls-Royce, immediately parking it where no cars were allowed, in front of the School Shop overlooking the playing fields. Bruce emerged already in his football gear and sat on the bonnet of the car to put on his football boots. Finally, Auntie May got out wearing a mink coat which reached almost to the ground like one of Bud Flanagan's. She also wore a magenta turban to match the car, and on it sported a huge and real diamond brooch.

This vulgar display of ostentatious wealth filled me with embarrassment and I slunk back to my study, later to be beaten for not cheering the school match. To top it all Repton won by three goals.

At the beginning of October 1939 I went up to Oxford. The Blackout had become a part of life, and the phoney war had begun. There was a general feeling of anticlimax. But I didn't go to Merton. Already the whole of St. Alban's quadrangle, in which was the top floor room I had chosen and expected to look out over Merton Field and Christ Church Meadow, had been occupied by the evacuated Ministry of Aircraft Production. Displaced Mertonians were put out to University College in rooms overlooking the High. I shared one with an amiable Classical Scholar from Mill Hill, Denys Wilde, the first of so many later to be shot down in the R.A.F.

Unlike my first day at Shrewsbury the atmosphere at Oxford was relaxed and civilized – at least for about an hour. Our room was quite beautiful, fully panelled with an ornate ancient ceiling bearing painted plaster crests, and reputed to have been occupied by Charles II.

As we were unpacking our things Denys and I heard noises from the next room which sounded like shots. On investigation this is what they turned out to be. Lying full length on the couch was a young man with unruly hair and a relaxed smile, wearing cavalry twill trousers and a hacking jacket.

'Come in,' he said hospitably. 'Help yourselves to some sherry.'

He continued to fire his Webley Air Pistol at the crests on his plaster ceiling, bringing down great lumps.

'What you doing that for?' I asked astonished.

'Are you a Vandal?' enquired Denys.

'No.' He grinned. 'An Old Wellingtonian. Must get some target practice in before the Huns get here.'

He picked up a box of long club matches and stuffed one down the barrel of the pistol. 'Switch out the light and watch this,' he commanded.

In the darkness he flung back the curtains and opened the window. Through the gloom we could see a bus-queue waiting on the other side of High in front of All Souls. Our host struck the end of the match on the window pane and fired a flaming missile in an accurate parabola. It landed on the target scattering the small crowd with alarm. He cackled with delight.

'Want to try a shot?' he asked offering us the gun.

But the bus arrived before we could respond. He shrugged, closed the window and the curtains and topped up our glasses. His name was Thursby-Pelham.

Later in the war, by then an officer in the Guards, he silenced a German machine-gun post in Tunisia, virtually single handed, doing some very nasty things to several of Rommel's army and thereby collecting a number of decorations. When I heard about this, it was clear they never stood a chance.

His room and schoolmate Chris Bulteel was a quiet contemplative soul except for a habit of playing 'The Emperor Concerto' at full blast on the gramophone in the early hours. This often brought up G.D.H. Cole from the room below, remonstrating that his writing of socialist tracts was being seriously impeded. The two Chrises apologized profusely and when Cole had gone pleaded with me to play the intro to 'Bugle Call Rag' on my trumpet. Bulteel and Thursby-Pelham were both reading History but in the annals of the War they made some themselves. Bulteel came back and the last I heard of him he was the headmaster of a school in Sussex.

My tutor in Physiology was a Fellow of Queen's called Dr. Carter. He smoked a large pipe and made kind remarks about my weekly essays which had titles like 'The Bundle of Hiss' and 'The Reticulo-Endothelial System'. But the real interrogators in the Anatomy Department were Solly Zuckermann, then doing research on monkey's gonads and female sex-hormones before he later joined the War Council, and Dr. Alice Carleton who terrified and shook me rigid when I took my first dissection viva. She had blue-rinsed beautifully coiffed hair, very blue eyes and a tongue capable of lacerating sarcasm and ridicule. I later became her house-physician in the Dermatological Department at the Radcliffe Infirmary. She then changed into a sweet kind woman of devastating charm.

We were each allotted in pairs to a particular part of a cadaver to dissect. There were eight dissections to complete each term. My dissecting partner was a small rather nervous girl called Janet Poulton. I immediately asked her to tea at Fullers in the Cornmarket, to sample the famed Cremonas at five pence each, but my tentative gropings for her hand under the table met with a swift rebuff, and I soon moved on to other targets as Pelham would say.

Janet worked intensely and efficiently at the first dissection which was the axilla and breast of the wizened body of a very old woman. The formalinized greasy brown dead flesh seemed to bear no relation to a once healthy human being. I read through the hundred odd pages in Cunningham's practical manual on the night before the viva having spent my time in that first week joining all three University political parties as well as the Union, because I had learnt they all had a dance each term. I got quite drunk at the Freshman's Blind. I also went twice to the cinema. One of the films had an actress in a small part whose name I did not know, but whose breasts and axillae greatly attracted me. She was in fact Rita Hayworth before she had become a star. I dreamt about her and was still an ardent fan by the time she made *Lady in the Dark* and *Gilda*. (My illusions were only eventually shattered over twenty years later one night in the Dorchester Hotel.)

I was therefore not in the best of mental or physical shape when Janet and I elected to take our first viva with Alice Carleton at the end of the week.

'Miss Poulton and Mr. Thorn,' she addressed us formally. She wore the crispest, most well-cut white coat in the department. 'Is this your dissection?'

We nodded. A long-shafted steel probe ending in a small hook came out of her pocket, held in a beautifully manicured hand. She poked about with it lifting up various structures. Janet answered all her questions, save one, with accuracy. Alice nodded approvingly. The blue eyes looked at me straight and true, and I was treated to a slow smile. The detail in Janet's performance had rattled me, and I felt a decidedly sinking feeling.

'And now let's see what you know, Mr. Thorn,' Alice said and lifted up a red length of tissue. 'What's this?'

I began to relax. All veins in the cadavers had been injected with a blue substance, and all arteries with a red. It was dead easy.

'An artery,' I answered confidently.

Alice's smile disappeared.

'What artery?' she asked irritably.

'Er . . . er . . .' I fumbled.

'Well, where is it?'

'In the . . . er . . . armpit.'

'Axilla!'

'Yes, I meant axilla.'

'Brilliant,' she said. 'What are its branches?'

'Well, there's one . . . er . . . that goes to er . . .'

'Names, names, Mr. Thorn.'

Suddenly it all seemed worse than Tombling.

'I . . . don't remember the names,' I said. Alice dived at another structure.

'What's this?'

'A muscle.'

'Yes, yes, but tell me its name, its origin, its insertion, its action and all the anatomical relations, its blood supply, its nerve supply . . . well?' she ended.

'I'm afraid I don't know all those,' I said.

'I'm afraid you don't know anything, Mr. Thorn. Have you done any studying at all for this dissection?'

'Oh yes, I've read it all through, but I . . . I didn't realize we had to go into this fantastic detail. I . . . I've been sticking to the general principles.'

'Mr. Thorn,' said Alice, 'anatomy is the study of fantastic details as you put it. You have to know everything. Every word in Gray's *Anatomy*. Every single word. Otherwise you could be a very dangerous surgeon. Go back to your college, and don't take your head out of your books till Monday morning, then I'll test you again.' She held out her hand. 'Give me your card.'

She wrote something in the first square. Here we go, I thought, 3% Thorn. But I was wrong. It was 0%.

I did as she said and went back to her two days later. The score this time was 80%.

'That's more like it,' smiled Alice. 'You see Mr. Thorn, you have illustrated an important general principle. Even idiots are capable of learning.'

Thereafter I treated every vessel, nerve, ligament and tendon, however small, with an intense and detailed respect.

Very shortly, the especially intensive course of study demanded of a medical student – lectures, labs, dissection, essays, tutorials, amassing facts, facts, facts into the small hours – became so heavy that there was precious little time for any of the more generally educative widening and amusing activities of Oxford. I had no time for games except occasional squash. The Junior Common Room, the Union Debates, the theatres and the Sheldonian saw little of me; except when my godfather, Malcolm Sargent, came down to conduct a concert. He invited me to the Green Room during the interval and introduced me to the soloist and leader of the orchestra. He stood, a dazzling figure in tails, talking with effortless wit and knowledge on any subject to the crowd of fans and autograph hunters, his free hand playing arpeggios up and down the arm of a glamorous sequin-sheathed young woman at his side. He seemed to inhabit a magic world far removed from Hitler's and even more from the anatomical intricacies of the brachial plexus and the movements of the elbow-joint. It was all part of the lure of show-biz which I knew could so easily subvert me. I felt there really was a nightingale singing in Berkeley Square.

Perhaps the scene made me determined to have at least some fun away from the books.

I went for an audition to recruit new members of the University Jazz Band grandly named the Bandits Club Orchestra, held in a rehearsal room over Taphouse's music shop at the end of Cornmarket. The band was run by the President of the Club, a first-year theological student, Bertie Moore, later to become a bishop. Bertie was almost as dapper and charismatic as Malcolm Sargent. There were four trumpet players as candidates for two places. The saxes had already been selected, notably Frank Dixon, the Senior Classical Scholar of Magdalen, who played wild but harmonically faultless extemporizations on a tenor-sax and could 'jam' indefinitely any twelve-bar blues. He owned the largest collection of 78s I have ever seen. After the war he ran his own recording studio and radio programme in Manchester.

I was a 'dots' man principally and luckily the brass were given a sight reading test. The first two players faltered and fluffed and Bertie soon gave them the 'Don't ring us, we'll ring you' treatment. The third was an extremely goodlooking young man from Christ Church, an English Scholar, Roger Frisby. He gave a very creditable rendering of a difficult bridge passage in 'I Got Love'. I followed this with the B passage in a chorus of 'Bugle Call Rag'. We were signed up, and the practice began, Roger on first horn and myself on second. Bertie dished out the parts of a new commercial number from Brons which must long since have passed into oblivion, called 'Hang Your Heart on a Hickory Limb'.

We swung into the four bars intro and first chorus. I blew as hard as I could. Bertie stopped us.

'I can hear the harmony far better than the melody line. You two change places,' he commanded Roger and me.

We did so.

'Now attack it,' ordered Bertie. 'I want it solid with bounce.'

When we reached the end of the piece, our lips were starting to feel that incredible flaccid pain which a succession of top C's can produce if you haven't practised for a long time.

'A bit ragged, but you'll do,' said Bertie.

And so I remained at the first trumpet desk, and Roger at the second for the couple of years that we played at College hops. We even did some semi-pro gigs at places like Woodstock and Abingdon, for a couple of quid each and a few beers. We had a stage show in the Taylorian Institute which was the second half of the performance of a play by Sydney Keyes called *Hosea*.

The next year I was president and the drain on our personnel by the war-effort gradually took its toll. Dennis Mathew on piano left to join the Navy and Bobby Glanfield, drums, went off to get killed in an armoured vehicle in the Western desert. But others joined us, notably Denys Johnson who was an old friend from Mr. Whitfield's house. He came from a really talented musical family who could boast a string quartet in its members, with his mother and two sisters, Sheila and Jill. Denys could play pretty well any instrument and his ability to learn a new one was rapid and phenomenal. One Thursday before a dance booked at St. Hilda's on the Saturday we learnt that Bill Darby, the trombonist, had been called up. Without hesitation Denys bought a new instrument from Taphouses, no doubt with resources from the Westminster Bank, his father being the manager of the main branch in Manchester. He dropped every other activity, changed his reed embouchure to a brass one and practised eight hours a day. On Saturday we played with a full brass section again. After all, 'In the Mood' is unthinkable without a 'bone.

That year we made wax recordings of two numbers 'The Maid's Night Off' and 'Wedding of Pocahontas' at the small recording studio in St. Giles and ordered a hundred Decca pressings. We actually sold over half of these to our university fans and I still have two scratchy ones. They sound pretty awful but at least still fill me with pleasant nostalgia if played after a bottle of Bollinger.

We also went up to the B.B.C. recording studios in Maida Vale for a programme that was broadcast later in competition with our Cambridge counterparts. The affair was hosted by Leslie Perowne, who disconcerted us on arrival in the huge studio by asking us if we wanted 'a split layout'?

As president I had to give an answer.

'No thanks,' I guessed.

'Good choice,' said Perowne and all the mikes were changed round and we were ready to go. Not, however, before Denys Mathew (who later was in the *Ark Royal* but returned to become a church organist), had managed to get a day's compassionate leave for the occasion, and had insisted on trying all the five grand pianos which were littered about. He finally chose a Bechstein but pronounced it 'a bit flabby'. Perowne informed him that Myra Hess had just made a recording on it.

'Lovely, lovely,' laughed Denys and played a few bars of a swing version of 'Jesu Joy of Man's Desiring'.

Our performance was not very good, and I fluffed a top C. But it all eventually went out over the ether two days after Pearl Harbor.

I don't think Roger Frisby ever quite forgave me for being first trumpet to his second but our time in the Bandits cemented a life-long friendship. It is questionable now if either of us could blow a middle range B flat; not that such an achievement would be appropriate for a Queen's Counsel regularly appearing at the Old Bailey, or a Harley Street doctor.

The summer of the fall of France still found us *in statu pupillari* and we shared our trumpet playing, our Glenn Miller and Count Basie records, punts on the Cherwell, and girls to go with them. But the war eventually grabbed him and Roger went off into the Merchant Navy.

He used to send me coded postcards to let me know his whereabouts. I remember one which said 'Saw Dopey Joe last week'. I doubt if the censor or the enemy knew 'Dopey Joe from Baltimo, He's always on the go'.

In the meantime there was no way of my escaping the Medical Course, even if I had tried. And so I obtained my first B.M. and a B.A. in Honours Physiology. For the rest I joined the Home Guard at Oxford, and did fire watching on the roof of the Pathology Department. The Blitz had gone by and no bombs fell very near Oxford itself, there being an erroneous belief that there existed a secret pact with the Germans, that if we left Heidelberg alone, they wouldn't touch us.

When I went home for truncated vacations, I became a temporary Air Raid Warden, Humphrey Perkins' School being a main Air Raid Post. When there was a warning I donned my tin-hat, bearing a service respirator on my chest, and ran down into the village blowing a whistle. What good it did, I shall never know. All around me was the unreal undisturbed sight of a sleepy country village. The sounds of bombs falling, and searchlights metronoming the sky over Derby and Nottingham fifteen to twenty miles away were like sheet lightning and the distant harmless rumble of thunder. Our little pocket of English peace-in-war was ready but never called to duty, though during the Battle of Britain we were convinced that the invasion would come, parachutists would descend and the panzers would grind up Sileby Road from the South. We played our wartime games but God knows what it would have been like if the Huns had succeeded.

Oliver Pell, the Chairman of the Governors, was the Chief Air Raid Warden and the Commander of the local Dad's Army. He was also a good cricketer. He received the yellow and purple warnings of approaching enemy bombers by phone from Air Raid Headquarters in Leicester. He passed them on to me via the phone at my camp-bedside in my father's study. Such is the incredible propensity of the British to regard anything, even death and destruction as a kind of sport he invented a code – in case of Fifth Columnists who might be tapping the line – a form of words which crystallized into phrases like 'Goering's just opened the bowling from the Vauxhall end'.

During the latter part of 1940, following our retreat from the now totally occupied Continent, a battalion of the Gunners were stationed for training in the village. Once when I came home for a few days I found a young officer had been billeted on us. His name was Ted Eveleigh. I think he was one of the few officers who escaped from Dunkirk, in spite of a leg injury, by walking up a gangway on to a ferry boat, commandeering a bunk and sleeping, no doubt fitfully, across to Dover. He had taken a law degree at Oxford from B.N.C. a year before the war, married the Hungarian Beauty Queen of Monte Carlo the next summer, wooing her successfully against stiff millionaire competition. While staying with us he studied regularly on most nights for the Bar Exam. He also had a fine singing voice and my father accompanied him on the piano in the drawing room to pieces from various operas. He charmed my mother completely and the presence of a real soldier in the house reassured her about the eventual victorious outcome of the war. Although he spoke with knowledge and authority in the same way as he does now as a Lord Justice of the Court of Appeal, he only once demonstrated his ability to pass judgements. As the crumps coming from Loughborough became louder and louder, he put his head round the drawing-room door and said 'I think the cellar is indicated.'

10 Front Office

Insurance men – and I include underwriters, brokers, claims assessors and loss adjusters – are not by any means the grey-faced beings of popular myth, even if they do tend to wear grey or grey-black suits and sit in austere City offices. They are an eclectic breed. They will assure your life for an astronomical sum, or insure any object or occurrence against any eventuality; a pair of shapely legs, or even fat ones, a pedigree Dobermann Pinscher, or that it will not rain on 23 October in Abergavenny. These esoteric covers tend to fall within the grey area of freak insurance. And grey is a colour to which insurance men are sensitive.

The Head of School while I was at Shrewsbury, Ronald Prentice, married Sonia Bowring, of the great insurance family and the sister of one of my closest friends Norman Bowring, who sadly was killed in a bombing raid over Germany. Ronald invited me to the Baltic Exchange where I was offered an expensive sherry by the senior partner. I sensed a certain stiffness in the conversation. We then went to the Underwriting Room at Lloyds followed by lunch in the august dining room. Ronald introduced me to a number of important people, all of whom were polite but not exactly welcoming. I noticed they tended to drop their eyes to my feet before looking into my face. As we sat down to lunch I felt uncomfortable. After the hors d'oeuvres I asked,

'There's something wrong, Ronald, isn't there?'

'Wrong?' he smiled, 'what *can* you mean?'

'Well, you look as if you're embarrassed about something; me in fact?'

'Not at all.' He started to eat, but his eye dropped momentarily down to the toe of my left foot which was protruding from under the side of the table. 'Why should I be?'

With a flash of intuition, my father's war-time admonition rang in my ears.

'It's my shoes isn't it?'

He looked at me with a pained expression.

'Yes,' he said.

I glanced round the room at the uniform black polished Oxfords under the other tables.

'They're suede! That's it, isn't it?'

'Grey suede,' corrected my host.

'Ronald,' I apologized solemnly, 'I really *am* sorry. I've embarrassed you acutely.'

Our wine was served for his tasting.

'I shall live it down,' he observed, nodding to the waiter. 'It's all quite bizarre. But you must be the first man to dine at Lloyds in grey suede shoes. Congratulations.' He chuckled suddenly. 'Do them good. You're also wearing a narrow tie.'

'My underpants are a preppy tartan,' I informed him, standing up as if to undo my trousers.

'For Chrissakes sit down,' Ronald hissed. Then he threw his head back and laughed. We continued to laugh intermittently throughout the meal.

'I promise you I'll never do it again,' I said.

'You won't get the chance,' he twinkled. 'And you'll have to be beaten after lockups.'

We have remained the best of friends all through the years. I haven't been to Lloyds recently and for all I know the aspiring young underwriter now sports jeans and kickers.

There is a much more relaxed atmosphere at the headquarters of the Entertainment Industry Department of the Fireman's Fund Insurance Company on Wilshire Boulevard, Beverly Hills. Dick Barry, the chief Underwriter, Scott Milne and Don Cass invited me to lunch recently at the office canteen. This turned out to be more like a five-star restaurant with a huge menu. The conversation was strictly about business, that is to say golf, drink and women. A few people were wearing ties. It was highly enjoyable.

At Pinewood Studios, there is a very lively bunch of chaps, part of the same organization, Ruben Sedgwick – whom I know well – Robin Hillyard, Peter Robey and David Havard. Robin plays cricket and golf to near professional standards, but his overwhelming charm hides a shrewd and professional expertise for gathering film insurance and assessing risks.

I have been with him on many locations where medical claims have arisen. He told me that a long time ago when he was very young and starting the job, he had to discuss a claim with the formidable producer Otto Preminger who was making a film in the South of France. Robin had arrived late the night before, and had been induced to tie one on by some of the cast and production company. The next day when he turned up for a very early appointment with Mr. Preminger, intending to impress on the producer the toughness of the Insurance Company's attitude, he was feeling, to say the least, somewhat 'pastel'.

'Mr. Preminger,' he began. 'I think I should tell you at the outset, that the Fireman's Fund takes a very serious . . .'

Otto held up his hand and fixed Robin with an unwavering stare.

'Mister Insurance Man,' boomed Preminger, with a voice full of menacing chunky gravel. 'I don't thing you're looging zo good.'

Fred Geddes, of Toplis and Harding, handled many film claims before he was superseded after his untimely death by the incomparable Jim Guild of E.I.A. Fred was a man of bulldog-like tenacity when on the trail of a claim during a film. He also could become highly emotional and irascible if he felt there was something fishy going on. When discussing with me in great detail the medical history and treatment of an artiste he would not hesitate to ring me up at 1 a.m. to have a recap. I was speaking to him daily and nightly through the huge claim on *Cleopatra*, and also seeing Elizabeth Taylor at least twice a week throughout her long incapacity at the start of the film, during which the elaborate set of Alexandria also disintegrated in the terrible autumn weather which struck Shepperton Studios. (A similar calamity took place when John Huston was making *Moby Dick* and the first mock-up of the great white whale disappeared over the horizon in a storm off the Irish Coast.)

Once, in Rome, Fred was on a hot scent over a claim which got him very agitated. We spent an evening going over and over it. Instead of my prescribing a suitable sedative, we had a drink at the Flora, walked down the Via Veneto to the Excelsior, had another, and then walked back to the Flora. I became aware that the process might continue indefinitely, so I steered him to the St. George for dinner. It was a bad choice, because one of the best restaurants in the town was not the place to go with Fred that night. His wrath had moved away from Cinecittà to Italy and Italians in general. He accused the head-waiter of not knowing how to cook spaghetti, and complained bitterly that the Asparagus Vinaigrette was too thin, too cold, and not swimming in hot butter. This was obviously his way of coming to decisions, because the next morning he was as bright as paint and settled the claim without a hitch.

Night work, fortunately, is not much of a feature of a film insurance practice, but owing to the time difference between Los Angeles and London, it can occur. I have a number of times picked up my bedside phone to hear on the line the voice of Dr. Morris Blacker, the Chief Medical Officer of the Fund. He is a delightful and knowledgeable man with an English wife, who went to Queen's College Harley Street, a long time before my daughters. I had recently examined Peter Sellers for a film and I remember the phone conversation went something like this:

'Is that you, Ron?'

'Yes.'

'Morrie here. How are you Ron?'

'Fine, thanks, Morrie. How are you?'

'Fine, Ron, just fine. I want to ask you about Peter Sellers.'

'Has something happened?'

'No. He's fine, just fine.'

I heaved a sigh of relief and changed the phone to my other ear.

'What's the problem?' I asked.

'Well, we've had your report on Peter, and everything seems fine, but we want to ask your opinion on what would be the effect on Peter if he were to fly five thousand feet up in a non-pressurized plane?'

It was a contingency I hadn't considered. I thought a moment or two.

'Ron . . . are you there?'

'Yes, I'm here.'

'Well, what do you think?'

'I didn't know he had to do any flying in this film.'

'He doesn't, Ron, he doesn't. But just supposing he took it into his head to do just that? What in your view would be the effect on him, and should we put a clause in the policy?'

I thought again.

'No,' I said.

'There would be no extra risk?'

'Not in my view.'

'If he went in a non-pressurized plane up to five thousand feet, you think he'd be OK?'

'Absolutely.'

'Hold on, Ron, hold on . . .'

I realized then from the sounds down the line that I was having a conversation with several people.

'Ron . . .?' Dr. Blacker's voice came on again.

'Yes, Morrie.'

'Are you prepared to guarantee that Peter Sellers will come to no harm in a plane?'

'If he should go in one?'

'That's right.'

'On medical grounds . . . er . . none.'

'You sound a little hesitant.'

'Only about the pilot and the plane. Not Peter Sellers.'

'Hold on, Ron.'

There was once more the muffled sound of discussion.

'Ron?'

'Yes Morrie?'

'We should all like to thank you here for your help and expert assessment, as the general on the ground, in this situation. We all appreciate it. Thank you Ron. Bye now.'

The line clicked off.

'Goodbye,' I said, put back the phone and turned off the light. I didn't sleep very well. There must be something to it all. In fact there wasn't. All went well with Peter Sellers, and the film. But then in film insurance everyone knows you can't be too careful. Especially with risks that might even come from Mars. There are millions of dollars at stake.

Accidents to artistes and resulting disability are automatically covered by the insurance policy. The examining doctor does not have to assess this risk but I have often wondered if a knowledge that dangerous sports are indulged in, or in the personality of the artiste which could make them accident-prone should not be mentioned to the company. Genuine accidents occur often enough during the course of a film and some productions seem to be plagued by them, particularly during the recent tendency of some companies to get artistes to do things which should properly be left to the stunt-men. *Moby Dick* collected a number and so did *A Clockwork Orange*.

Janice Rule, who looks ten years younger than her years, came in to see me wearing a black leather tunic trimmed with mink over trousers, and carried a formidable handbag. She had a charming smile and a husky New York accent. At the time mugging in the Big Apple was frequently making the headlines, which prompted me to ask,

'Do you carry a gun?'

'No. My husband does.' She laughed. 'He won't let me. He says I'd hold it the wrong way, and kill myself.'

I wasn't entirely convinced.

Sir Ralph Richardson always seemed indestructible.

'Came on my motor-cycle, my dear fella. Much faster. Can park the damn thing almost anywhere. Always been a motorcyclist. Killed myself dozens of times.'

The insurance doctor enjoys no such insurance protection except that provided by himself. An examination can carry its own hazards. Visits to locations in tropical or sub-tropical zones require a load of inoculations themselves carrying risks and some are very uncomfortable. So far I have escaped any of the more unpleasant conditions such as Loa Loa or Hookworm Disease.

I did on one occasion ask the instructing insurance company to provide me with a short policy covering me against injury, when I learnt that their previous doctor in a foreign city had been knocked out cold by an artiste at the outset of the examination – the doctor had refused to risk repeating the performance. Needless to say I wasn't issued with a policy. My examination went off without any fisticuffs but I must admit I wished the rubber tubes on my stethoscope had been double their usual length.

I also find it slightly intimidating when a lady star insists on the examination being carried out in the presence of her boyfriend, husband, protector or whatever.

I went to examine Jayne Mansfield in a rented mews house in Belgravia. Somehow she had put in a fairy princess bed with a flimsy draped canopy up to the roof. She exposed herself with a million-dollar smile and stared me in the eyes during the whole time I listened to her chest. This was disconcerting but quite bearable. What unnerved me was behind me. Micky Haggerty, whose head nearly reached the ceiling, was lifting up and down his bar-bells with suitable grunts of effort and occasional growls throughout the procedure beyond the end of the bed. He sported a very proprietorial expression. I was very glad of the strictures imposed by the General Medical Council concerning professional conduct and discipline.

Marlon Brando usually has a protective female companion at his bedside and recently I examined Jack Palance in a hotel while his wife slept off her jet-lag on the other side of the bed.

The cast medicals for *Lawrence of Arabia* had either been forgotten or left too late for them to be carried out in London. I had to go to Amman in Jordan to do them.

I think most people have had the experience when they feel that a series of mishaps, accidents, near-misses, are beyond the laws of chance; a feeling that someone 'up there' or 'down there' is out to get us. My friend Neville Main believes that the deity is constantly administering little shocks and warnings if we get too cocky. He refers to the Gentleman as Fred.

The atmosphere of premonition really started just before I left for the Middle East. During lunch at home in the flat, there was a heavy storm. The children were young enough to be frightened by the violence of the thunder. I told them that no lightning ever strikes in the centre of London. The conductor was a broad copper band right outside the window. Immediately after my observation there was a brilliant flash and crackle down the conductor combined with an instantaneous ear-blasting thunderclap which sent us all under the table. So much for Daddy's reassurance.

The next day my second wife Halina and I took her car for a motoring trip to Switzerland. A dozen miles south of Arras we passed the scene of an accident. After a weak protest that I was on holiday and not going to stop, I pulled up, took the First Aid Kit out of the boot and ran back to where a small crowd had gathered. Proclaiming that I was '*médecin*' I found an old bald-headed man lying on the grass verge where he had been carried. There was a sizeable laceration on his scalp, the blood already clotting well. He had been unconscious and was just coming round. There seemed to be no other injuries. The old boy started to shiver. I put a dry dressing on the wound and told the gawping spectators to fetch a rug, a coat or even a car carpet from somewhere to keep him warm against shock, and send for an ambulance. My Salopian French patois was met with blank stares. At that moment a motor-cycle arrived and the uniformed driver, who appeared to be a member of the French equivalent of our St. John's Ambulance Brigade, dismounted. Bristling with officialdom he pushed me roughly aside, removed my dressing, and with none too clean hands manipulated the scalp wound presumably to determine its depth.

'*Voila!*' he exclaimed.

All Tombling's efforts to instruct me in French Prose Composition vanished into the summer air.

'You bloody idiot,' I exclaimed. 'All you've succeeded in doing is re-start the haemorrhage, infect the wound, and make his condition decidedly more dangerous.'

The man drew himself up and glared at me belligerently.

'*Anglais*,' he said. '*Allez vous en.*'

At that moment the ambulance arrived.

'*Merde!*' I retorted and left them to their Gallic devices. As I reached our car, I tripped getting into it. My back 'went' and pain shot down my left leg.

I was driven by Halina to our booked first night stop at a château hotel near Dole. We arrived in the middle of a French wedding reception, through which I was assisted painfully up an enormous staircase. Halfway up was a macabre life-size tableau of a bride and groom.

With difficulty I had a bath, got into bed and ordered a bottle of champagne. Halina was intrigued by the figures at the wedding standing in the garden. She took three photographs of them from our window.

I passed an uncomfortable night which was not helped by the sound of revelry which continued into the small hours. The next morning while attempting to put on my sock, I stumbled against the side of the antique bed, barking my shin, and cursing this time in three-per-cent German. Then to my relief I found my back pain had disappeared. The fall had provided a gratuitous manipulation.

As we were paying the bill, when the receptionist enquired whether we had slept well, I replied that the noise of the wedding reception had lasted a long time, and kept us awake. She raised her eyebrows.

'What wedding reception, Monsieur?'

'The one yesterday.'

'But there was no wedding yesterday.'

'Of course there was,' said Halina. 'I took some photographs from the window.'

'You must be mistaken. Here is your receipt.'

We went off in the car. We discussed her extraordinary attitude. Halina then told me that when she had had dinner alone, as I was in bed, she learnt that the figures on the stairs were of two people who got married some seventy years ago and had tragically drowned in the little lake at the back of the château on the first night of their honeymoon.

'So we imagined the whole thing?'

'Of course,' said Halina. 'It explains everything.'

'Balls,' I replied somewhat colloquially.

At Evian where we were staying I had the photographs

developed. There were three charming views of the garden taken from the bedroom window – trees, lawns, flower-beds – but no figures.

As soon as I returned to London, I was rung by the insurance company and asked to go to Amman. I left the next day. At Heathrow I was approached by a smiling semitic character with a package, which he said contained morphine 'for some very sick people' in Jordan and as I was a doctor, it would be much easier and much better if I took it through the customs at the other end. A sheaf of five-pound notes were barely hidden in his hand.

'Nothing doing,' I said.

He shuffled off but I wondered how he knew who I was.

At Amman I was ensconced in the best hotel opposite the Roman amphitheatre. The place, though comfortable, had a musty brimstone smell about it. I received several phone calls, which were intermittently cut off, with the production company and David Lean, the director. There had been a change of plan, and everybody was already on location at Aqaba on the Red Sea some three hundred miles away through the desert.

'We've got a little two seater plane to fly you down,' I was told. I was at that time at the height of my aerophobia and the invitation immediately conjured up a single-engined plane crash or at least a forced landing in the desert. For the second time that day I said,

'Nothing doing.'

'Well, we'll have to lay on a car for you tomorrow, but it'll be a long uncomfortable trip.'

'I don't mind that,' I lied, and so it was arranged.

The next morning, an attractive looking middle-aged American woman with a camera slung round her neck came up to me in the foyer.

'I'm Mildred McCargur,' she said. 'Sam Spiegel's P.A. You're Dr. Thorn?'

'Yes. How do you do?'

She thrust out a red-nailed bejewelled hand.

'I'm coming in the car with you to Aqaba. Sam's in his yacht down there so he can keep tabs on the shooting schedule. The picture's going to be one honey of an expensive one!'

The car was a sturdy old Buick with a sturdy old Arab driver. On the front seat beside him was a Jordanian soldier in full kit, carrying a machine pistol.

'What's he for?' I asked.

The driver smiled a knowing Eastern smile.

'Bedou,' he replied and shrugged.

Mildred and I got into the rear. Soon we left the sparsely green

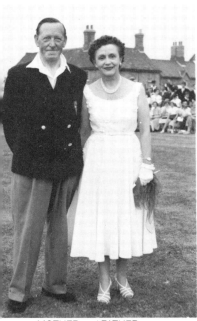

MOTHER and FATHER
'the most intelligent thing I ever did was to
choose these two people for parents'

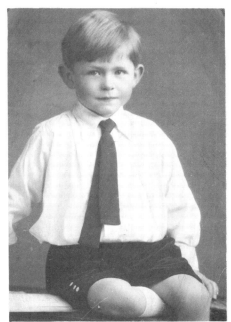

AGE 4½
'Ronnie mustn't get a swollen head'

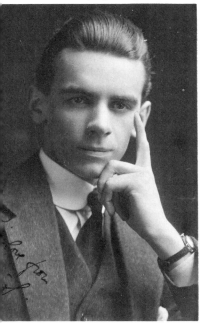

GODFATHER:
Sir Malcolm Sargent 1920

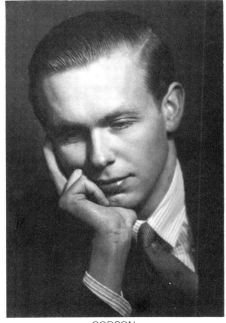

GODSON:
Author 1947
Photo Fayer Camera Portraits

Oxford University Bandits Club Orchestra — 1941

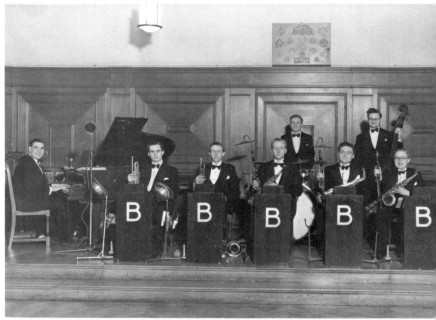

At the piano: Dennis Mathew. Front row: (left to right) Roger Frisby, Author, Denys Johnson, Ivor Jones, Frank Dixon. Back row: Bobby Glanfield, John Boothby

Photo Gillman & Soame, Oxford

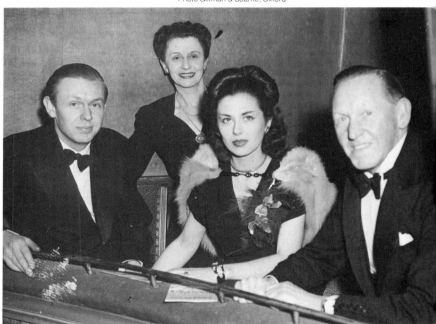

Author and family at the first night, Mountain Air, Comedy Theatre, 1948

Location, *The Full Treatment,* the Riviera

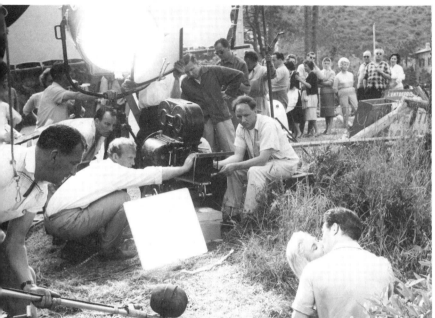

Author (right of floodlight), Val Guest (left of floodlight) (far right) Diane Cilento, Ronald Lewis
Photo Val Guest, Columbia Pictures

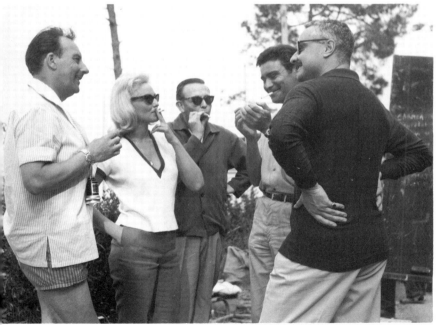

(left to right) Val Guest, Diane Cilento, Author, Ronald Lewis, Michael Carreras
Photo Val Guest, Columbia Pictures

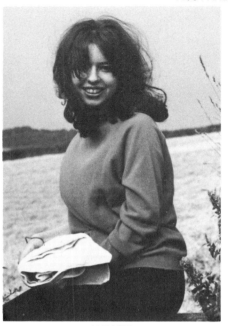

AMANDA
Photo Ronald Scott Thorn

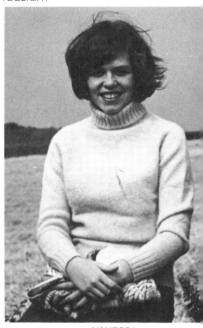

VANESSA
Photo Ronald Scott Thorn

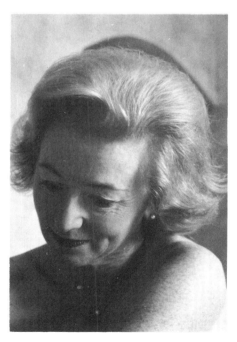

MURIEL: 'She came in through the windo
like Elvira in *Blythe Spirit*'

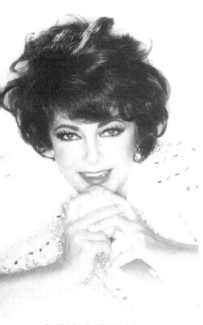

ELIZABETH TAYLOR
Photo Norman Parkinson Camera Press London

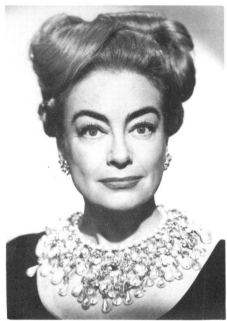

JOAN CRAWFORD
Photo Camera Press London

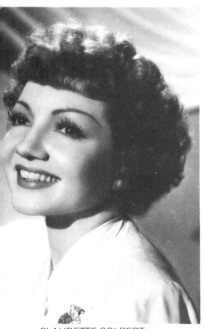

CLAUDETTE COLBERT
Photo Camera Press London

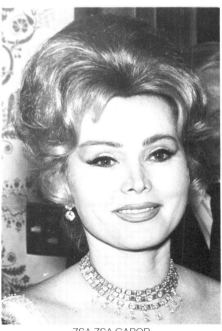

ZSA ZSA GABOR
Photo Julian Wasser Camera Press London

'Even less to be paid for the privilege...'

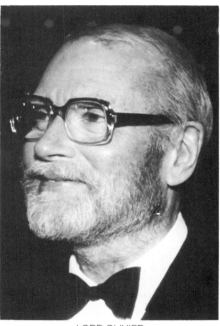

LORD OLIVIER
Photo Ray Hamilton Camera Press London

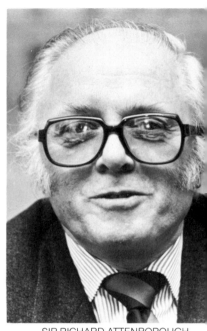

SIR RICHARD ATTENBOROUGH
Photo Camera Press London

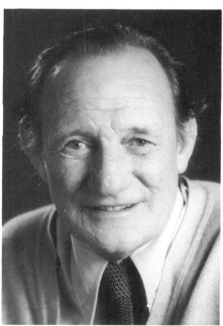

TREVOR HOWARD
John Timbers Camera Press London

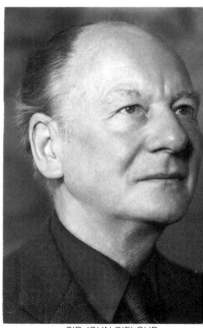

SIR JOHN GIELGUD
Photo Yevonde Camera Press London

'Not averse to playing tricks on the medical examiner...'

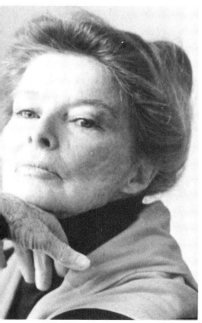

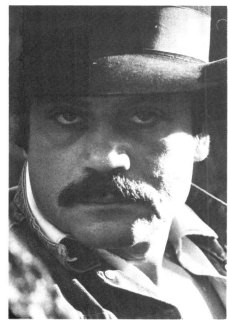

KATHARINE HEPBURN
Photo John Bryson Camera Press London

OLIVER REED
Photo Brian Aris Camera Press London

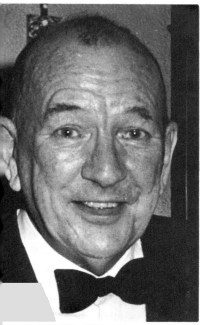

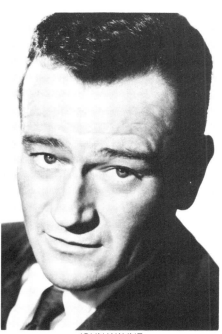

NOEL COWARD
Photo Brodrick Haldane

JOHN WAYNE
Photo Camera Press London

'…A sense of humour, if not of the ridiculous, is essential sometimes both on and off the consulting couch…'

THE STRASSE (Harley Street)

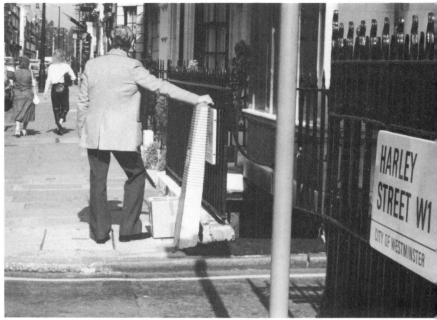

Diagnosis: L5/S1 prolapsed disc with right sciatica

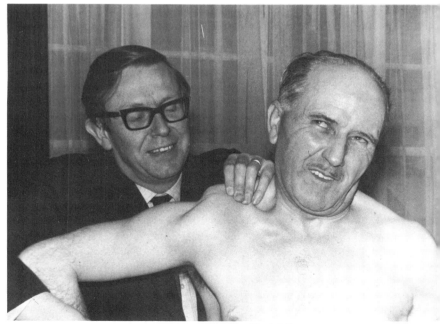

Author with unidentified victim

Photo ALP Jeffery

'An unsuitable case for treatment'

irrigated areas south of the city and were very quickly amongst the wide rolling landscape of sandy desert. The road became a dusty bumpy track. The heat built up intolerably and a kind of stupor finally vanquished Mildred's chatter. In less than an hour she had told me her life and love story at least twice.

The scenery changed as we reached the place where a blue and purple vista of cliffs and plateaus stretched into the distance with incredible silent, timeless beauty. Mirages of mountains and lakes came and went and twists of sand rose in whirling clouds for a second or so and then subsided.

The driver stopped the car and an ice-box was opened. Coca-Cola was gratefully drunk. I got out with Mildred to stretch my legs. She exposed a whole roll of film exclaiming ecstatically and then re-loaded her camera in the relative shade of the back of the car.

'As good as Colorado?' I asked.

'Much, much better. This is simply weird.'

After the break, we drove on, and almost immediately the driver slammed on his brakes and we came to a jerking stop. In the centre of the road was a low pile of rocks. The soldier got out and stood at the back of the car, his weapon at the ready.

'What is it?' whispered Mildred.

'Bedou,' said the driver. 'They block the road. You can't drive round it in the sand. They kill you, take everything they can, push the car off the road, take down the rocks and disappear. In no time you're just a mound of sand at the roadside.'

'But I can't see anyone,' said Mildred, getting out of the car.

The soldier motioned her back in. The driver said,

'When they do arrive, don't let them see your camera. It's an insult to take a picture. Just get down and keep quiet.'

We did as we were told. Several minutes went by and then they were there, just beyond the stones. Three camels and three robed riders. No one moved. The silence continued. The heat increased. This is the time, I thought, when Peter O'Toole should arrive, and talk us out of the situation. Unfortunately he didn't show up.

Abruptly the soldier opened fire spitting up the dust at the base of the stones. The Bedou did not move. He gave another automatic burst. This time the three camels turned away and in a second it seemed they had been swallowed up by the desert.

The soldier walked forward with the driver and they shifted some stones making a gap in the pile. Then they ran back, and jumped in the car. We shot ahead, accelerating madly and didn't slow to a normal speed for five minutes. The soldier smiled and so did the driver.

'My God,' gasped Mildred.

'No,' smiled the driver. 'Not Allah. Just Bedou.'

The basic location site at Aqaba was built like a compound, the atmosphere being of a base camp for an assault on some high mountain. It was presided over not by Mr. Spiegel, who stayed in his luxurious yacht offshore, but by David Lean, arguably the most intelligent, knowledgeable and talented film director in the business. Talking to David on any subject is a stimulus and an education. On the job he is the supreme perfectionist.

Believing that the comfort of the troops is important in winning any battle, he had organized dozens of well-equipped trailers for the stars, artistes and chief personnel. I was allotted a commodious one for the night I stayed there. I carried out all the examinations in a well-equipped medical room where the location doctor did a clinic twice a day. The air-conditioned canteen provided first-class food with steaks and other supplies flown in from time to time.

All these lush conditions contrasted with the morning selection of Arab extras who scrabbled and fought for tokens for work outside the gates. What they were paid a day I do not know but the delight on the faces of those who were chosen told its own story.

My assignment completed, I decided to take an extra day away to do some sight seeing. I wanted to visit Jerusalem. Unfortunately I had not been told I would need two passports, since Israel at that time would not accept one that had a visa in it from the Hashemite Kingdom of Jordan.

Peter O'Toole suggested I went to Beirut instead on the way back and gave me the names of several nightclubs. In the event I never went to any. The trip in the car back to Amman was uneventful, but when I reached the hotel I found an invitation to dinner from Dr. Khouri, surgeon to the King. He and his wife ran a private hospital where he performed brain and thoracic surgery, and she gave the anaesthetics.

He had a pathological museum containing interesting specimens of massive gallstones, huge bladder calculi and other pickled tissues which he had removed from important patients all named and classified. What disconcerted me was that patients were wheeled through this somewhat macabre collection on their way to the operating theatre.

Khouri and his wife were hospitality and courtesy itself. I had been warned of the massive number of courses which were served at Arab feasts. I didn't get the traditional sheep's eye but I had to have second helpings of everything. I discovered the hazards of the Bedou and air-travel were as nothing to this ordeal. When I returned to my hotel afterwards I really felt I should die from hyperdistension.

Through a very hot night of this suffering I remembered the similar predicament of Ted Eveleigh. Just after the war he was sharing his flat with Frank Brandt, a solicitor. They were cooking for themselves. One night they treated each other to a generous curry. They were just sitting down to recover from their blowout when the phone rang. It was an old army colleague, Fitzgerald-Moore, a stickler for protocol and etiquette, and incidentally the Billeting Officer at Barrow-on-Soar in the War, who had selected our house for Ted's billet. The conversation on the phone, I believe, went something like this: 'Ted? Fitzgerald-Moore.'

'Hello. How are you?'

'What's happened?'

'What do you mean?'

'Well, we're waiting dinner for you and Frank, and you're over half an hour late. Mother's very upset.'

Ted suddenly remembered the invitation. There was no way out with Fitzgerald-Moore, an authority on Debrett and Burke's peerage.

'Frightfully sorry, old boy,' said Ted. 'We've been badly held up. All apologies. Be with you in twenty minutes.'

Gasping with bloated stomachs, Ted and Frank squeezed into their dinner-jackets, got a taxi and made it to the flat in Westminster. Their hostess accepted their apologies graciously.

'Doesn't matter at all,' she said. 'It's only curry. I know that's one of your favourites, Ted.'

The two guests managed to eat thoroughly but slowly. I believe conversation was somewhat limited, and eventually came to a standstill when they were pressed to second helpings.

In Beirut after a short flight with Air Jordan in an overloaded old Dakota, where the other passengers rushed from side to side, regardless of the barefooted hostesses handing out sherbet, to point out to each other familiar landmarks, rocking the plane, we cleared the mountains it seemed by ten inches. Fred in the sky was obviously out to get me.

In Beirut I spent a whole morning buying presents for the family. After about ten cups of Turkish coffee, an obligatory custom in each shop, I staggered back to my hotel and went to bed for the rest of the day. I couldn't estimate the number of grains of caffeine I had absorbed but could count my pulse-rate. It was a hundred and thirty. I shook like a poplar leaf for several hours. It was time to go home. I believe a bomb exploded in the foyer, a few minutes after I left.

But my battle against the powers of light and darkness had not ended. The day after I was back in London, I was driving to see a case along the Marylebone Road. Opposite the London Clinic I became suddenly blind in one eye due to a retinal vein thrombosis. The condition cleared up in six weeks, but I took it as a salutary warning, especially for an insurance doctor. It also happened on my fortieth birthday. But I have not yet decided whether this was chance or intentional.

11 The Cutting-Room

Because of the war I did my clinical training at the Radcliffe Infirmary, Oxford. Most London teaching hospitals were evacuated to various parts of the country because of the bombing. We collected St. Thomas's.

It was an immense advantage to have such additional teachers like the physicians Sir Arthur Hurst and Professor Ryle (of Ryle's tube); the orthopods Trueta (of secondary wound closure), Girdlestone (of the Girdlestone hip) and Seddon (of the peripheral nerve grafts). The war effort brought together neuro-surgeons like Cairns and Pennybacker, the ophthalmologist Ida Mann, Mackintosh and Mushin in anaesthetics, and McArthur in tropical diseases. Chassar-Moir, J.D. Flew, and John Stallworthy made innovations in obstetrics and gynaecology. All these luminaries were in addition to our own physicians A.M. Cooke and Hobson. There was a strong home pathology, bacteriology and haematology team with Robb-Smith, McFarlane and Florey who was developing Fleming's work on penicillin. The dosage was originally measured in Oxford units. Sinclair was revolutionizing the knowledge of nutrition. Chain was indulging in flights of fancy about carcinogens; I have already mentioned Zuckermann.

Nuffield money was pouring in and clinical material was drawn from most of the south of England. The mantle of Osler lay over everything. It was difficult to imagine a better place for studying the 'art'. Knighthoods and Nobel prizes were distributed later. The sheer concentration of so many original minds was itself awe-inspiring. The atmosphere was electric and exciting. Things were developing at enormous speed and the clinical students were expected to work in the same manner.

Among my own contemporaries were Dennis Melrose who invented the first artificial kidney machine. John Butterfield is now knighted, and Regius Professor of Medicine at the other place, Cambridge, and Master of Downing College. At Merton were Derek Wood who is now a Professor of Pharmacology at Leeds, and Gordon Beckett who is a consultant endocrinologist at the Royal Free Hospital.

In spite of the tremendous advances in medical knowledge and technology, the scanners and the computers of today, there still remain with me the fundamental truths in the aphorisms bequeathed by my teachers of that time.

'The commonest diseases occur most frequently.'

'Any condition will either get better, get worse, or stay the same.'

'In ninety-nine cases out of a hundred if you feel well, you *are* well.'

'In ninety-nine cases out of a hundred, if you do nothing, the patient gets better.'

'In ninety-nine cases out of a hundred, the correct treatment *is* to do nothing.'

Because it grows at extreme biological speed and taps the resources of the whole body it was once said that,

'The most malignant tumour of the uterus is the human foetus.'

'The ultimate totalitarian dictator is the human baby.'

This is probably why man, with his special upbringing, is the most dangerous organism in the animal kingdom.

The intensity of the clinical course was exhausting and almost completely excluded any other activity. A surgical dresser or medical clerk in the wards not only had to take histories and examine the patients in detail, but in the face of opposition by ward-sisters who rationed the time of access to *their* patients. Students were regarded as nuisances. As with the anatomy we had to know every minute detail of the patient's condition and life and be prepared to discourse on a case either on a ward-round or present the case at a clinico-pathological meeting not only to one's fellow students, but one's teachers and any illustrious guests who might attend. As a method of learning it was incomparable, but it was an awesome ordeal.

Surgery had a dramatic lure, and assisting at an operation a sought-after privilege. Strangely, I never felt squeamish about the blood and the observation of living tissues being cut, removed, sewn-up or transposed except on one occasion. Sight of the surgical battlefield was one thing, the sound of bone saws another, but the sense of smell really got to me.

At my first thoracic operation where ribs were resected and the moving lungs and heart exposed, cautery was used to seal off multiple small bleeding points. The odour of burning flesh and the thin spirals of blue smoke proved too much for me. I felt an overwhelming nausea and faintness. The whole operating theatre started to shimmer and swim like a mirage. I remained conscious long enough to hear the surgeon say calmly,

'Get him out someone before he falls across the table.'

I recovered in the surgeon's room feeling ashamed and mortified. At the end of the operation the surgeon grinned at me kindly over a cup of coffee.

'Gruesome business, isn't it Thorn? But you'll soon get used to it. You can get used to anything in time.'

In time I did.

Surgeons of course vary in their attitudes to beginners and are given a god-like respect by the nursing staff. A few indulge in a sarcasm which can be devastatingly humiliating.

I remember much later when I was qualified and had to give an anaesthetic to a very heavy, bronchial individual, given to taking large quantities of alcohol. These factors require the dosage of anaesthetic to be increased to produce the necessary depth of unconsciousness. The skilled anaesthetist gets them quickly through the early stage where the patient struggles and fights. I was having no luck at all. It was in the days of open ether and I had two porters holding the patient down, while I sweated behind my mask to get him under. After a very long while the surgeon got tired of waiting and came into the anaesthetic room. He surveyed the scene with expressionless eyes and then enquired casually, 'Are you winning, Thorn?'

Professor Finlay, a fiery tall thin Scotsman, provided us with great amusement in the V.D. clinic. He was of the old school who considered correct treatment of such conditions required, in addition to the exceedingly painful course of mercury injections, a discourse on morality and the sins of man.

He would line up the male patients in front of him, stripped to the buff, shivering with fright and at times the none too warm room in the outpatient clinic.

'Well?' he would ask the first in the line. 'How did you contract it, you wicked snivelling creature?'

'D . . . d . . . don't know sir.'

'Never been with a woman, I suppose?'

'No sir.'

'Ach, I see. Well did you play between her thighs?'

'Well . . . er . . .'

'Bend over. This is going to hurt.'

And he would jab the long intramuscular needle deep into the quivering buttock. The patient frequently howled in pain.

'Stop that noise,' Finlay would rasp. 'You've got eleven more of them to come. Return next week.'

Most of them did, but some were never seen again.

One patient, a farm labourer, stated, after the usual denials, that he must have caught it from the seat of a plough.

'Aye,' said Finlay, his eyes narrowing. 'Then it'll have been the hoar frost, nae doot.'

The needle went in inexorably.

At the beginning of the clinical course at the Radcliffe, I moved out of college and went into digs at 18, Beaumont Street. It was an approved university lodging run by Dorothy Protheroe. I had a large room on the first floor with a delightful view of the Georgian houses opposite, mostly occupied by dentists. There was a small iron-work balcony from which I could look down to the beautiful clock on Worcester College. It was strategically placed for the hospital, and hence within easy reach of the nurses' home, that supply of pretty uniformed damsels, the students' consolation for the exhausting academic programme. Further up the street was the Ashmolean with its Elgin Marbles where the Slade School of Art was temporarily housed, another source of female companionship of a different order; but more interestingly, number 18 was less than a stone's throw from the Playhouse, where I went to a performance each week, and near the Randolph bar.

About this time the Americans had come to the new Churchill Hospital at Headington; a surprising notice had appeared on the students' board at the Radcliffe. It was suggested that we should offer some Anglo-American hospitality by showing some of the nursing staff from across the Atlantic round our colleges. I quickly entered my name on the list.

Some days later two gorgeous girls arrived for tea. Their uniforms were as glamorous and their cosmetics as flawless as the creatures one had seen in many American movies. I was determined not to let them down and showed them round Merton.

I was not at all put off by their comment about Mob Quad, the oldest quadrangle in Europe.

'Look at it all Fran,' exclaimed one blonde beauty. 'This place is so old it's rotten.'

'Sh . . .!' said Fran noticing Gavin Townend, a third year scholar, subsequently Professor of Classics at Durham, who was sitting in a deckchair in a corner surrounded by books. Without looking up, he raised his boater and replaced it.

'Who's that?' whispered Blondie.

'Er . . . that's the captain of the college,' I said. 'He's very much older than he looks.'

Gavin repeated the performance with his straw hat.

'Can you imagine that, Fran?'

We moved past Gavin on tiptoe to the Fellows' garden, where there is an elevated terrace on what was once the ancient town wall. We gazed across Merton Field to the long avenue of trees of the Broad Walk. I was in my stride now and gave the nurses a graphic description of the great events of history which had certainly not happened there. It was King Blank fighting the Battle of Blank all over again, and consisted of a hotch-potch of everything I could remember about Agincourt, Bannockburn and Culloden. I knew it had gone down well because when I had finished, Blondie repeated again,

'Can you imagine that Fran?'

Fran looked over the wall with misty eyes,

'I sure can. I sure can,' she replied wistfully.

I remember Fran had a pair of legs like Zizi Jeanmaire.

Some of the rooms at Number 18 were let out as theatrical digs to the permanent members of the repertory cast at the Playhouse and also to more well-known visiting actors and actresses. I found the atmosphere extremely congenial. Breakfast in the basement was often a delight when troupers like Muriel Pavlow, Rosalie Crutchley, and Roberta Huby appeared in dressing gowns or revealing negligees to eat the wartime sausages and the rationed butter and margarine.

These were all diversions which leavened the hours of midnight oil studying the heavy tomes of Price's *Practice of Medicine*, Bailey and Love's *Textbook of Surgery*, and Russell Brain's *Diseases of the Nervous System*.

My room was also a haven for non-medical friends who had left to fight the war and descended for short leaves. Equipment and khaki or RAF blue uniforms littered the place and often I had the room filled with sleeping beer-filled snoring forms on the bed, the couch, in the chairs and on top of the desk. As someone in a reserved occupation, I felt this supply of free accommodation was the least I could do. Many of them showed me their ailments and discussed ways and means to deal with the complications of their camp or station peccadilloes. I pontificated and then steered them either to the Radcliffe or recommended they made a clean breast of things and went to their MO's on return to their units. There were some great reunions and noisy parties. When they left I cleaned up the mess, played some Fats Waller or Benny Goodman to soothe my frayed nerves and prepared for the next onslaught.

Inexorably the day of reckoning drew nearer. In the war situation you were allowed two attempts at Finals; in peacetime as many as you could afford. The three main sections, Medicine, Surgery, and Obstetrics and Gynaecology all had to be passed at the same examination and could not be split up like the Conjoint diploma of MRCS, LRCP. Down in one was down in the lot. A failure at the second attempt meant 'out' and into the Forces. The assignment was a tough one but Jack Roberts, Sheila Jones and I decided we would have a go at the Finals – just as a practice run three months before it was strictly necessary. It was a risky ploy. After the two weeks of gruelling papers, long cases, short cases, and multiple vivas, to our surprise we all passed in June 1944 while the news of D-Day and the flying bombs was coming in.

It was an exhilarating feeling to read the notice pinned to the Pitt-Rivers Museum doors and read one's name on the list. 'The following candidates have satisfied the examiners in the Schools of Medicine, Surgery, Obstetrics and Gynaecology.' We were doctors but the euphoria was tempered by Dr. A. M. Cooke's remark when I managed to land my first hospital job at the Radcliffe itself.

'Now you can really start to learn, Thorn.'

Before I took it up – it was a mixed appointment, children and skins, which meant my chiefs were Finlay and Alice Carleton – I had two weeks' leave.

I decided not to waste this precious opportunity. I telegraphed my girl friend Sarah Murchison, a Wren I had pounced on for the last dance at a Services Ball held at the Randolph earlier in the year, which I had gate-crashed. She was on leave with relatives in the Western Isles of Scotland. I went up on the train and she met me at the Kyle of Lochalsh. She had black hair and violet eyes which surpassed those of Elizabeth Taylor.

Impetuously and theatrically I undid the small brooch she was wearing, given to her by my rival, her former boy friend in a Highland regiment, and tossed the brooch into the swirling waters from the ferry as we went over the sea to Skye. She slapped me on the face. I kissed her and asked her to marry me. Then she laughed with one of the most attractive gurgles I had ever heard, and agreed to the proposition.

On the way back we stayed with her parents in Edinburgh. Her father was a Wee-Free Minister and the atmosphere of non-drinking, non-smoking sanctimony in the manse gave me my first misgivings. I played two very long games of conversationless chess with Sarah's father whom I could not believe had sired such a lively attractive daughter who was a ball of fun and an accomplished Gaelic singer. After the ordeal she crept into my bedroom, and produced a half-bottle of Scotch and twenty Players. We leant out of the top floor window smoking and drinking, and later removed all traces of our sins.

At least that was what we thought, but mother had found clues, and I departed under a definite cloud. Although the engagement was made official in the *Scotsman* and *The Times*, our enforced separation, while I did my job at the Radcliffe and Sarah went back on duty, had its effect. The engagement was broken off before Christmas, the ring returned. I wonder where she is now.

When I had finished the job at the Radcliffe I took up my second obligatory hospital appointment at Bournemouth. But in the break between the two I did a short locum for a GP in Suffolk. The change to a country practice after all the hospital years would be a stimulating challenge. I remembered as a boy going out in Dr. Gray's car on his rounds at Barrow flanked on the rear seat by Marie and Eva. A car-boot containing a brace of pheasants, a home-cured ham, jars of chutney and jam and half a Stilton cheese at the end of the day seemed a pleasant way of doing business. At last, trained but green, I was to test my skills in the field so to speak, using eyes, ears, hands and nose, without all the hospital technological backup, X-rays and laboratory tests. I felt like an old prospector or frontiersman. Though not required to do rounds on a horse like Doc Holliday, I was going at last to have the use of a car, with the privilege of unlimited petrol, when rationing had taken nearly all civilian vehicles off the road.

Dr. Bailey-Britton had slipped a disc. Unable to get about, he was lying on a board on his bed with painful sciatica. His instructions were simple and to the point.

'You do two surgeries a day, and dispense the medicines. There's the red cough-mixture and the black cough-mixture, a tonic containing strychnine – so watch the dose – and use Senna for constipation, and Whitfield's ointment for skin. You'll find a red cross on some of the notes. This means they're flaming nuisances and nothing wrong with them. Keep these characters at bay by giving them a bottle of what I call 'Mist. Nausea Co.' It's harmless but contains a lot of Asafoetida. Makes them stink to high heaven, and socially unacceptable for days.'

'Yes, sir,' I said, wondering if all the high-flown biochemistry and pharmacology I had so recently absorbed had really been necessary. It all sounded so basic.

'By the way, my partner – sleeping partner I call him – will do alternate night calls with you. You're on tonight. All right. Off you go. Try not to kill anyone.'

'No sir,' I said and went towards the bedroom door.

'Oh, salary. Five pounds a week OK? Cash?'

It seemed to me a generous reward.

'Thank you sir.'

I opened the door.

'One more thing,' the voice behind me made me turn again. 'There's an old tobacco tin on my desk. Any letters which arrive where the stamp has not been franked, steam it off and put it in the tin. Got to be economical you know.'

My first two surgeries and rounds of visits went off without any difficulties. I dispensed the medicines and put them wrapped and secured with pink string and sealing wax on the hall shelf to be collected and had my supper. It was starting to snow outside. I went to bed feeling tired but exhilarated.

I was called out three times that first night. A nosebleed which had stopped by the time I found the place; a breech delivery at a farmhouse, an acute appendix which took a lot of phoning to get into hospital in Ipswich. I got back to bed at 6 a.m.

I started the next day exhausted and went through the same routine. The car broke down once, and I sprained my ankle in the snow. I was just on my way to bed, thankful not to be on night call again, when the phone rang. It was the partner in the practice. He sounded most affable as he introduced himself and added an invitation to sherry sometime in the near future.

'Oh, by the way, old boy,' he added as if it were an afterthought, 'I've got a spot of chronic sinusitis. Don't want it to flare up in this weather. I wonder if you'd mind doing the night calls.'

'Oh,' I said. 'Of course. Certainly.'

'Splendid fellow. Thank you. Goodnight.'

I did the next six nights on call without a break. At the end of this period I was looking decidedly older. Bailey-Britton remarked on my appearance. I told him the reason why I wasn't getting much sleep.

'Typical, typical,' was his comment. 'I told you he was a sleeping partner. Nothing wrong with his sinuses, lazy old bugger.'

I went to bed and slept twelve hours.

But I hadn't finished my association with the other member of the practice. He gave me the promised sherry, but the social contact did not entirely remove my resentment.

Two mornings later, after I had put the local prep-school in quarantine for measles, I was called to see the wife of the local squire. She was in fact a patient of the partner, but he, as usual, was otherwise engaged.

The woman was in her early sixties. I was shaken by her appearance. She was bright yellow, in severe pain, and had a rigid abdomen. Observing the courtesies, I rang the partner from her home and said I was going to admit her to hospital.

'What on earth for?' he asked tetchily.

'Obstructed common bile duct. Maybe a sub-phrenic abscess too,' I said.

'What absolute bunkum. She's got a mild hepatitis.'

I swallowed hard.

'When did you last see her?' I asked.

'Oh, I don't know – week ago. Wasn't too bad then.'

'Well she's an acute emergency now.'

There was an ominous silence.

'See here, young fella,' came the answer. 'When you've been in practice for a decent time, you'll realize you mustn't panic . . .'

'I'm not panicking, but she'll have to go in for an immediate operation.'

I was shaking with a mixture of anger and doubt. Was I making a fool of myself? A groan from the bedroom clinched it. I said, as calmly as I could,

'If she isn't sent to hospital I will not take the responsibility for the outcome.'

There was a very long pause.

'All right,' came the answer at last. 'I'll be straight round to see her. But if you're wrong I'll get Bailey-Britton to send you packing.'

Later in the day the partner admitted the patient to the local nursing home and a surgeon came out from Ipswich. I was just having my lunch about 4 p.m. when the partner's by now familiar voice came on the line. The tone was unctuous and patronizing.

'Thorn?'

'Yes.'

'Not a bad bit of diagnosis. You're learning fast. The operation's on.'

'Good,' I said, feeling that all the responsibility was now in his court. But I was wrong.

'Just one point, old boy. I wonder if you'd mind assisting?'

'But she's your patient.'

'I know,' he said. 'Fact is I've never relished the operating theatre. Always feel a bit dickey. I'd be extremely grateful if you'd stand in for me. I've told Willie you'll do the job and I've fixed John Mortimer for the anaesthetic. All right? Cutting at five o'clock.' The phone clicked off.

The nursing home had twelve beds, a sparkling white new theatre, and was quite efficiently run by the matron and three nurses. I was quite impressed because private nursing homes in those days before BUPA and PPP had very mixed reputations.

But when the surgeon opened the squire's wife's abdomen a fountain of pus under pressure shot up to the ceiling.

''Fraid she's gone, Bill,' said the anaesthetist.

The abdominal wound was quickly closed and the patient returned to the ward. Afterwards the partner joined the surgeon, the anaesthetist and myself for coffee in the matron's room. I was left out of the conversation. Abruptly the surgeon frowned.

'Well? Who's going to inform the coroner?'

Four pairs of eyes looked at me unblinkingly.

'Coroner? What's the coroner got to do with it?'

'Death on the table always has to be reported. Surely you know that?'

'Yes,' I said, recalling the tedious lectures on Forensic Medicine and Public Health which seemed then so far removed from reality.

'You'll have to give evidence at the inquest too,' said the partner.

'Need I?' I asked.

I suddenly felt surrounded and under attack. Why should I have to do all the unpleasant jobs?

'It wasn't my fault,' I began.

The surgeon put an arm round my shoulder like an uncle with his favourite nephew.

'Ever been in this situation before?' he asked quietly.

'Er no sir, but . . .'

'You see you have to learn not to worry about it. You have to try and forget the distress to the husband.'

'It won't bring her back, will it?' I heard my voice rising emotionally.

'You have to learn that too, lad,' said the surgeon.

A sickening sensation of lethargy and defeat overcame me. I put on my coat and picked up my bag and left the room. I recognized for the first time that medicine like a lot of other things wasn't all cricket.

The Royal Victoria and West Hants Hospital Bournemouth had about three hundred and fifty beds. A number of regular consultants had been taken into the Forces. A number of retired ones came out of hiding and other elderly gentlemen appeared from distant parts. A particularly lively octogenarian was Colonel Whittamore, late of the Indian Medical Service. He was put on to supervise Casualty and Minor Ops. He still maintained his old priorities and treated the nurses like coolies. In the mornings, while the new casualties sat in line awaiting his attentions, he never started until he had finished reading *The Times*. He was rather deaf and to entreaties from the Casualty Sister to start the clinic, he would reply:

'I see Burmese Rubber's down another two points. What? what?'

We residents had to give gas for him while he incised boils and whitlows with fearsome despatch. On Thursday afternoons he did six circumcisions. He approached each mother carrying her already screaming son with the warning,

'Now see here, mother,' he would bark. 'I shall only do this operation on medical grounds, not religious ones, understand?'

After a brief examination, he would often say,

'Nothing wrong. Get out. Next.'

The operating list was thereby substantially cut down, if not the infant.

There was an RSO Max Minchin, an Australian who had taken

up Medicine late, having previously done Forestry down under. He was studying for his Fellowship, eventually obtained, and has recently retired as the senior surgeon at Perth Hospital, Western Australia. He was an excellent operator and tireless doctor, seemingly requiring no sleep at all. I was a new House Surgeon and Casualty Officer, and later HP and RMO. I learnt a great deal from Max.

There was Bert Ostrovsky from Edinburgh, and Ainslie Eggeling, the resident medical officer, and Harry Williams from St. Andrews. This completed the Scottish contingent. Jim Fisher was from Cambridge and Alec Walker from St. Mary's. It was a small team to run a big hospital, and largely inexperienced. We had very little sleep and were all on caffeine to keep ourselves going. I calculate that we packed in as much experience in a year as we could normally have gained in five years in peacetime. Remembering all the things we were asked to do, and did, often now brings me out in a cold sweat. But somehow we were never responsible for a medical or surgical tragedy.

The food for the residents was disgusting. I was paid three pounds ten a week. We had one half-day off which usually started about 5 p.m. Harry Williams and I often got off duty together and went down to the Norfolk Hotel bar. Harry had a biting wit, but his weakness, like many Scotsmen, was that he was a competitive drinker. One evening after a session on the town, when we returned the worse for wear, he was on night-call for the medical wards. They called him out. I was horrified but not surprised to read the next day his nocturnal note on one patient written all over a complete page in a large barely legible scrawl:

'She's no breathing so weel.'

I took out the page and repeated the remark in ordinary writing. Harry signed it later.

All of us conducted a running battle with the hospital secretary, an efficient but self-important man without a sense of humour. We pinched the paint which had arrived to redecorate his office and used it on our own quarters working through the night. He was apoplectic when he saw what we had done and gave the impracticable order:

'It'll all have to come off again.'

But his office remained in its pre-war dingy state.

As a final attack we went too far. Jim Fisher and I collected all the toilet rolls, including the ones from Matron's room, the nurses' home, outpatients and Saul's private loo. We cut a stencil for the rotary Gestetner duplicator and faking Saul's signature, printed on each sheet of paper the patriotic legend,

'Wartime Economy. Please use both sides.

By order of the Secretary. Gordon M. Saul.'

It was a dirty trick but led to an explosion of mirth throughout the hospital. Saul never forgave us. The senior physician, Tom Robson, got the thing in perspective. He said to me, 'When are you lads going to grow up?'

About this time an incident occurred which foreshadowed my future medico-legal career, though I had no inkling of this at the time.

I was called to Casualty in the early hours to find a policeman had accompanied an old lady nearing her seventies who lived with her older husband in a caravan site north of the town. She and her husband had been in the habit of befriending a homesick young GI from the American army camp nearby. Apparently he had gone berserk, killed the husband with a hatchet and beaten up his wife.

She was in severe shock, had been unconscious and had bruises all over her, but no more serious physical injuries. I don't know what prompted me to do it – perhaps a suspicious or an overimaginative one-track mind – but though there were no obvious signs around her vulva, before admitting her to the ward for treatment, I took some high vaginal swabs. I went to the path lab and made smears on some slides and stained them with Methylene Blue, and Haematoxylin and Eosin for good measure. I don't think even then I expected to see anything, but under the high-power of the microscope I found three spermatozoa and one doubtful one.

I didn't tell the police then, waiting for confirmation from the consultant pathologist next day. If I was right it meant not only murder but rape. The pathologist confirmed my findings.

A few days later an American Medical Corps colonel in full uniform arrived at the hospital and asked to see me.

'Are you the guy who thinks he can see spermatozoa on some slides you have here?'

'That's right sir,' I said. 'I can see them. So can the consultant pathologist.'

'Is he here?'

'Not at the moment. He'll be in this afternoon.'

The officer looked at his watch.

'I can't wait till then,' he said and then smiled invitingly. 'Maybe you could give me the slides and I can take them away to have our lab check them?'

'I'm sorry sir,' I said. 'But they belong to the hospital. I can't let them be taken out. You're welcome to look at them in our lab here.'

He scowled perceptibly.

'OK. Lead the way.'

I conducted him to the path lab, produced my slides and offered him the stool in front of the microscope. He stared at it for a second and then turned to me.

'What the hell is this? You mean to say you haven't got a binocular microscope?'

'No,' I replied. 'But this oil immersion is perfectly OK.' I focused the object-piece on one of the slides and manoeuvred it to bring one of the spermatozoa showing the head, centrepiece and the long tail clearly and incontrovertibly. 'There,' I said. 'I think you'll find that more than adequate.'

He took off his cap and sat on the stool and looked down the eyepiece. After a slight pause, he asked,

'You call that a spermatozoa? It's so badly stained it could be a thread of cotton.'

'With a head and a tail?'

'Hell, these are just artefacts. Show me the others.'

I did so.

'I guess this is very doubtful evidence.'

'The consultant pathologist doesn't think so.'

He got up.

'OK,' he said. 'You let me take these slides and I'll get them properly checked.'

'Sorry, Colonel,' I said putting the slides away. 'Nothing doing.'

'Say, Doctor, er . . .?'

'Thorn.'

'Dr. Thorn. How long have you been qualified?'

'Just over a year.'

'A year? Do you know how long I've been in this business?'

I was really getting steamed up.

'Seventy years?' I said.

He put on his cap, hiding his balding head.

'Look, if those slides are your evidence, I tell you, they won't stick.'

But they did. Some weeks later I was called to give evidence at a court martial at the American camp. The 'courtroom' was in a prefabricated hut. The Judicial personnel were highranking officers. They sat at the table, drinking I presume Coca Cola, and smoking. The prisoner lounged in a chair chewing gum. I was disconcerted by the movements of the cross-examining counsel who shot questions at me, from the front, sides and even from behind me.

But I stuck to my guns and the court martial, in spite of the apparent laxity, reached a fair and just conclusion. The prisoner was found guilty of murder and rape. He was shipped back to the States pending definitive sentence.

I was just leaving the camp when the Colonel came up to me

with a wide grin and shook me by the hand.

'Well done,' he said. 'I'd like to have you on my side in a fight. Good luck.'

I went back to the hospital but not without a call at the Norfolk for one of Harry Williams's malt whisky specials.

By the end of 1945 when peace had broken out we were a much more sober and experienced lot. We had still to do our war service. In fact the day I reported for my medical for the Armed Forces at the Military Hospital near Millbank was the day Japan capitulated. The examining Colonel took one look at the X-rays of my Salopian hip and passed me unfit for military service. He banged a rubber stamp on my file.

I left the Royal Victoria at the beginning of 1946, jobless and undecided what to do. Under Robson's encouragement, he told me to take my MRCP and become a consultant as soon as possible. But it didn't work out like that.

12 'Zoom'

Though I had written some short stories at school which no magazine publisher would accept, and scribbled away at some verse, which I ambitiously sent to *Horizon*, to collect rejection slips but also courteous letters from Cyril Connolly, it never occurred to me that I might be able to write a play. The chances of having one performed anywhere, let alone in the West End seemed totally remote. Roland Maule in Coward's *Present Laughter* convinced me of the utter futility of such effort especially in wartime – until I met Justin Power.

He was ten years older, and had been invalided out of the New Zealand navy in the thirties. He came to England and was employed by the American marketing research firm A.C. Nielsen and Company which was stationed in Oxford. He was an ardent theatre-goer and seemed to me, as a raw student, a polished man of the world. He had read every play I had ever heard of. Our common interest might have stopped there, had he not suggested we write a play together. I told him I thought it was pointless to write things which would never be performed. He then surprised me with the remark, 'But I know the Chairman of Tennents and

Binkie Beaumont, the Managing Director. They'd certainly read anything I put in their hands, and if they liked it, they'd produce it.' H. M. Tennent at the time had five productions running in the West End. In a flash I saw my name in lights.

On the basis of 'It's not what you know but who you know', I thought perhaps we might have a try.

In my room at 18 Beaumont Street, we sweated away in the small hours. At least I did. I found I was doing most of the work. Justin would contribute what I considered some extremely witty lines.

I showed our first effort about undergraduates to my father, who laughed it out of court. Undaunted Justin submitted it to Binkie, who replied, 'A jolly little piece about nothing in particular'. Our second effort I showed to Joan Marion, a West End actress and film artiste who was billeted at Barrow with her husband, Nap de Rouet (in peacetime a wine importer) who was a Squadron Leader at the new RAF aerodrome at Wymeswold. Joan patiently and very kindly tore the play to shreds. Our third attempt called *Roast Beef and Chewing-Gum* was a topical fantasy about the Americanization of Britain which my father was persuaded to produce for the Old Students Dramatic Society. Just before Christmas Justin managed to get one of the de Grunwalds to come up from town on a very foggy night to see it. He made one or two mildly encouraging remarks which prompted me to send the script to W. A. Darlington, the drama critic of *The Daily Telegraph*, whom I knew was an old Salopian and who had written an article entitled 'Where are the new playwrights?'. Sadly, according to his lights, I was not one of them. I received a letter back from him that ended: 'You may be a playwright Mr. Thorn, but there's nothing in this rigmarole which leads me to think so. I am sure you should stick to medicine.' This was a sentiment which was echoed repeatedly by my father who thought I should not in any event be wasting my time writing. He then dropped the bombshell which started to sever my friendship with Justin.

'You can't plagiarize like you do anyway.' Picking up a script he quoted a dozen lines and told me from which plays – mostly by Noel Coward or Frederick Lonsdale – they had been taken. I remember going hot and cold at the revelation. I taxed Justin with the accusation and we had a blazing row. We had just completed a modern Passion Play called *The Man in the Market-Place* which I went through with a toothcomb and deleted all the lines which I discovered had been cribbed from Dorothy L. Sayers. I didn't send the script anywhere and Justin and I parted company.

But the writing bug had bitten deep. While at Bournemouth I sent two very short humorous stories to *London Opinion* and got them both published, being paid three guineas for each. I immediately sent off a third but the editor sent it back with the salutary comment, 'Sorry. Not *this* time.' Fair enough, I thought but I have been in print and received money for my efforts. Therefore I was a professional writer. I thereby acquired an incurable chronic infection. When I have time, I promised myself, I'll write a play on my own.

After leaving Bournemouth in January 1946, having stayed on as RMO for six months following my RAMC rejection I decided to take Robson's advice and try for my Membership of the Royal College of Physicians, a *sine qua non* for a consultant appointment. I persuaded my long suffering father to stake me for a year's postgraduate course in London and furthermore lend me his Hillman Minx. After all, as a doctor, I could get petrol coupons, and he couldn't.

I found a bed-sitting room in Barkston Gardens, Earl's Court, got out a pile of new textbooks and began attending lectures and ward rounds again. But after a month or so of diligent study my interest was diverted by London and the bright lights. I saw every play in town from the gallery, and went to every cinema. I also ran into Roger Frisby again, now demobbed and studying for the Bar in a bed-sitting room in Bloomsbury.

We met frequently for beers in pubs all over town. Out of this my second adventure in writing collaboration began. But it was a very light-hearted one, and we knocked off a mock-serious textbook on beer drinking called '*They're Open!*' long before Stephen Potter used a similar style and format and scooped the pool with *How to Win at Games Without Actually Cheating*.

We felt our book needed some pictorial lift. On a visit back home, through Christopherson, who was a friend of my father's and the head of the Leicester College of Art, I was put in touch with Neville Main, his one-time pupil and by then a professional artist and illustrator. Neville and I immediately found we had the same sort of humour and rapport and a deep friendship was struck up which has lasted to the present day. We were both Leicester-shire men. I was born in the north of that county of eccentric rural pursuits, and Nev in the south. He came from Peatling Magna, a village of less than a hundred souls. I often wondered what was the population of Peatling Parva but Nev had been strangely reticent on the point. Nev produced a series of brilliant line illustrations for the book.

I continued to send the script out, even after rejection by eighteen publishers.

Then, in an August number of the *British Medical Journal* I saw an advertisement by a Swiss doctor, offering free board and lodging in return for lessons in English. I posted off a letter immediately and had a quick answer inviting me to go. In his reply was the germ of an idea which was to mature and proliferate. He wrote 'I will you hospitality offer, and my wife will give you a good kitchen. We will all make expeditions to the mountains mit the bicycles.'

I took the car and motored through France. At that time there were few cars about and even fewer cigarettes. I soon learnt that twenty Players Medium Navy-cut would procure a full tank of petrol, a simple meal, and if so minded, a girl for the night. On the way to Switzerland I stayed in Paris as a guest of the de Dampierres, whose daughter in 1938 had stayed with us at Barrow to perfect her English. I was to go to her home the next summer. But that was 1939. By 1946 she was married to a diplomat and was living in Ankara. She wrote me saying Maman and her brother would be delighted to see me. Elie, the son of the Comtesse – who regarded anything that had happened since 1939 as a shocking irrelevance, including Hitler – had been in the Resistance and spent some time in the concentration camp at Belsen. He took it upon himself to give me a conducted tour of Paris from mid-day to beyond midnight. We sat in the sun on the inevitable Champs Elysées and he explained to me that the French like to see and be seen which accounted for the constant parade in front of us. I suppose, like most people, Paris bowled me over. I was entranced and captivated.

After we had done the Louvre and les Invalides, Elie insisted on giving me a gastronomic lunch in a small restaurant – where did all the food come from in these places at a time of great shortages? – and finally took me to the Folies Bergères in the evening. When we came out, he asked me casually, as if offering a cigarette, 'And now Ronald, perhaps you would like a nice goerl?'

'Well . . . I hadn't . . .'

'I mean something *spécial, très gentil*. One has to be delicate and selective in these things, yes?'

'Well, yes,' I said.

'Come along my friend.' He gave me a knowing Gallic smile. 'It is necessary to start with the very best.'

It was an offer I couldn't possibly refuse.

We arrived at the famous *Cent vingt deux*, Rue de Provence. A correctly dressed maid let us in.

'*Montez, messieurs*,' she smiled.

We walked up the beautiful curved staircase. At a corner she put her finger to her lips, opened an elegant door and we slipped inside what appeared to be a cupboard. I heard someone go down the steps on the other side.

'You see,' explained Elie, 'no customer here is ever allowed to meet another one. That would make this socially impossible.'

The door opened and the maid conducted us up to an elegant little salon and small bar containing genuine Louis Seize furniture. Madame, a couturier-dressed woman in her fifties, welcomed Elie with open arms. I was introduced and we sat and exchanged pleasantries, and drank some cognac. Like all civilized business meetings, the matter in hand was not immediately referred to.

'*Monsieur le Comte*,' she addressed Elie. 'I am afraid Jacqueline is not here tonight.'

Elie held up his hand.

'*Merci, madame*, tonight I am very tired, but my English friend here . . .'

'*Ah, oui*,' she smiled, and I was treated to a comprehensive glance of professional appraisal. She squeezed my biceps. I felt like a dog at Crufts.

'What is your special pleasure?'

'Well . . . I . . .' I said.

'*Alors*,' said Madame. '*Choisissez, Monsieur*.'

'I will help you,' said Elie. Madame opened another door and Elie and I followed her.

It was quite a large room. About a dozen girls in various costumes and stages of undress froze in a kind of tableau, all bestowing on us discreet expressions of invitation. The ladies of the bedchamber were all incredibly attractive. I smiled back inanely and fleetingly met the eyes of one or two. It was an *embarras de richesses*. How could I select one, without offending all the others? I felt myself blushing. Outpatients was never like this.

'*Choisissez*,' repeated Madame.

I raised a limp hand, and as if sticking a pin in a map, pointed at random to a sloe-eyed brunette in the front row. She came forward provocatively on her high heels.

'Bravo,' said Elie. 'Exactly the one I would have chosen.'

The girl and I went up in one of the lifts. It was a sumptuous room with a sumptuous bathroom. She gave me a thorough clinical examination worthy of Professor Finlay, then bathed, almost scrubbed and then dried me. We returned to the bedroom and another maid brought in champagne in a bucket, opened the bottle and poured the glasses. I paid her. My companion prompted me to double the tip.

We were left alone and I had a French lesson and learnt many new words, few of which were in old Tombling's vocabulary.

Afterwards I was conducted back to Madame's little salon, flushed and dazed.

'OK?' asked Elie.

'OK,' I said.

'I have paid,' he reassured me and bade Madame goodnight. When we emerged into the street, I said,

'Look Elie, I can't let you pay like this.'

'You are my guest,' he said.

'But how much . . .?'

'That does not matter. Another time,' he shrugged.

'I expect the amount was enormous. The champagne alone . . .'

He suddenly looked angry.

'Champagne? You should never buy champagne in a place like that! It's very inferior stuff.'

He called a cab, but by the time we reached his mother's flat off the Avenue Victor Hugo, he had regained all his charm and composure.

The next day I was on my own. I had a very sedate lunch with the Comtesse and then sallied forth once more to observe the manners of the town.

I was still totally bemused by my experience of the previous night. I sat at one or two pavement cafés unwisely drinking brandies. Each café seemed to take me nearer to the Rue de Provence. I thought of Rolande Raimbaud, for that was her name, with obsessive excitement. My sexual inexperience had been exploded like a Roman candle. But it was more than that. Professional it may have been, French it undoubtedly was, but the delicacy, the charm of my seduction fired me with extravagant puerile romantic fantasies. As the brandy warmed my stomach, my heart beat with a tender fervour. Ridiculous, I told myself, you can't fall in love with a tart! She's probably been with half a dozen men since you, already. So what? I built illusion upon illusion, piled Pelion upon Ossa. So long as she liked me more than the others. Cognac was a potent aphrodisiac. To hell with it, wasn't this what Paris was all about? The day was so beautiful. Why should I not enjoy it to the full? As I stood up and paid my *addition*, the Place de L'Opéra shimmered in the sunlight like a Monet or Pissarro. The attraction was irresistible, my desire unquenchable. I crossed the road mindless of the hooting vehicles. Doctor I might be, but underneath I was still a simple English country boy, a passionate fool, out of his depth, and hell bent on amorous adventure, whatever the cost. Distantly I heard my mother's voice 'You'll pay for it, Ronald'. In one sense she was of course absolutely right but my finger didn't waver as I pressed the bell-push in the Rue de Provence.

I knew the drill now and asked to see Madame. She looked faintly surprised.

'So soon Monsieur? *O, la la!*'

'I wonder,' I said, 'if I could take Rolande out for the day?'

'*Ah, pour se promener?*'

'*Oui.*'

'*Et la nuit aussi?*'

'*Bien sûr, Madame,*' I replied firmly. I must have sounded like a millionaire.

'*Attendez, Monsieur le docteur. Asseyez vous.*'

Her eyes continued an amused appraisal while I lowered myself into the Louis Seize bergère and she made a brief call on the internal phone.

'Rolande is *occupée* at the moment, but if Monsieur would care to wait, eveything can be arranged. Champagne?'

Elie's warning was still in my ears.

'No thank you,' I said.

She wagged a finger at me.

'Monsieur is learning, yes?'

I smiled back.

'I hope so.'

She laughed attractively.

'Come,' she said. 'You cannot wait here. As it happens, the house physician has just finished his round.'

The phrase didn't sound the same as at Bournemouth. 'You can talk together until Rolande is ready.'

She led me through one of the six doors of her little salon into another room. A well-dressed man in his fifties, drinking Perrier Menthe, stood up and we were introduced. The door clicked to expensively behind Madame.

Doctor Vincent proved a great conversationalist. He explained in some detail and with equal pride his daily visits to *Cent vingt deux*, making it sound like an appointment as Physician to the Royal Household. We discussed VD in all its aspects and he questioned me closely about its prevalence in England. It rather reminded me of a Finals Viva. Apparently I passed with an alpha plus.

The door opened and a smiling Rolande appeared. She looked absolutely delicious. She was dressed in a simple but chic chiffon dress with matching gloves, handbag and shoes. There was no jewellery, no tell-tale gold crucifix on a chain round her neck, no other tarty insignia. I was entranced. Dr. Vincent kissed her hand. Rolande pecked me on both cheeks like a sister, slipped her arm through mine, and we went down the stairs and out into the Paris afternoon.

I had parked the Hillman in a street behind the Madeleine and she chatted happily while directing me to her flat off the Boulevard Haussmann which she shared with another girl, who fortunately was not in. The place was simply furnished in a French provincial style and there were dozens of photographs of her family, and of herself as a child and at her confirmation. She told me she was thirty and trying to save money to study Fine Art at the Sorbonne. We drank a lot of wine and she made a recommendation for a restaurant for the evening. She disappeared to change for this event, and only when she appeared in a black sheath dress with a daring neckline, and provocative side-slit skirt, elbow length gloves with a diamanté bracelet, a fur stole, and high-heeled sandals which gave to her gait an unmistakable swing, could one possibly imagine she was anything but an expensive *demimondaine*. The very one Elie would have chosen, I reminded myself.

Where we went or what we ate I cannot remember but I drank far too much and on returning to her flat I dropped into a comatose slumber and didn't wake till the sun was blazing through the windows. So much for my idyllic night of love.

Rolande and her friend Denise were sitting in their *peignoirs* at the table drinking coffee. I joined them with a head like Bottom the Weaver. They ignored me while I recovered. Then the enormity of the escapade hit me, as I remembered that I had neither informed Elie nor the Comtesse that I would be out for the night. It was unforgivable, inexcusable behaviour. I shaved hurriedly with Rolande's tiny razor and cut myself twice. I ran a comb through my hair, but the mirror refused to reflect anything but a startled scarecrow. I dressed hurriedly.

'I must use the phone,' I announced.

'*Pas de téléphone*,' replied Rolande. 'There is a *cabine* on the corner.'

'No. I'd better go. Where is the car?'

'I put it in the garage for you. Here is the *billet*. All paid!'

'*Comme les Americains, les Anglais sont tous boirées*,' said Denise.

'Look, I have to go immediately. How do I get to the Avenue Victor Hugo?'

Rolande produced a street map and I worked out the route. Fortunately I wasn't very far away.

I kissed Rolande. She looked much older than I remembered.

'*Au revoir, chérie*,' I said. '*Merci mille fois.*'

I made for the door.

'Ronnie!' said Rolande. The 'R' had an attractive guttural quality, but the voice was hard and her expression grim. '*Tu n'a pas payé.*'

She handed me a slip of paper. Every detail of our evening's expenses was meticulously recorded, including tips. At the end came a large sum billed '*Service*' and another one which said '*Pour la maison*'. It was a formidable total.

I took out my wallet and Rolande counted the notes as I put them on the table. I was a few thousand francs short.

'*Eh, bien . . .?*'

'I'm terribly sorry, I just haven't any more,' I stammered.

'*Merde,*' said Denise. '*Vous n'êtes pas un chentleman.*'

'I will come to the bank with you,' said Rolande.

'That's no good, I haven't an account here, but I promise you I will come back and pay what I owe you.'

'When?'

'When, when I get back from Switzerland. Really I will.'

I produced a half empty packet of Players for her which she put on a shelf.

I was thankful I still had a quarter of the sum I had brought to France in an envelope at Elie's, but I needed that – and more – for the rest of my trip. I stood miserably shifting my weight from one foot to another and looking like Herbert Marshall who in most of his films at some point seemed to have the line, 'Oh, what a fool I've been!'

Then, to my surprise Rolande smiled, shrugged and kissed me.

'I do not believe you, Ronnie. But it is not the first time this 'as 'appened. *Au revoir.*'

She pushed me towards the door, and I stumbled down the stairs.

It was about 10 a.m. when I reached Elie's mother's flat. He opened the door, his face pale with a mixture of anxiety and anger. He let me in. I felt it best to make a clean breast of everything. 'I understand absolutely,' he said. He made a sign and we tiptoed towards his room. On the way we were brought up abruptly by the appearance of the Comtesse. Elie spoke to her in rapid French which was too fast for me. She cut him short and addressed me directly.

'*Monsieur,*' she said. '*A votre chambre!*'

I felt six not twenty-six. Inside my room I stood quite still and listened to the sounds of Paris coming through the window. What could I do to make appropriate amends to my hostess? Elie provided the solution. He came into the room, looking stern, and then grinned broadly putting an arm round my shoulders.

'So you have found out, my friend, what everyone finds out. Paris is not a city. It is a love-affair. And it is for life.'

I smiled back, relieved at his attitude.

'Maman,' he said, 'is very upset. She has been up all night worrying about you. I had great difficulty in persuading her not to get the *Sûreté* out to make a search. I rang *Cent vingt deux* and discovered what you were up to. I take part of the blame. Now, sit down, and I will dictate a letter.' He produced some crested notepaper, and a bottle of ink. All that was missing was the quill pen. In French worthy of the diplomatic corps, I wrote a letter of apology to the Comtesse. He put it in an envelope, and sealed it. 'You had better make yourself more presentable while I deliver this.'

He left the room. I had a hurried bath, and put on my 1939 grey chalk-stripe double breasted – and suede shoes. Elie returned.

'Maman will receive you now. Whatever she says I will do the talking. Then you will offer to do something for her. She was in Paris throughout the occupation and just managed to remain in the flat. Our cars were commandeered. She longs to go to Versailles again. You will take her in your car and bring her back. Then all will be forgiven.'

A little later I conducted the Comtesse down to my father's Hillman Minx. The old lady was made up to the nines, and was wearing a large flowered hat and a faded lavender flowing dress reaching down to her delicately laced booted feet. She carried a large parasol with a long carved silver handle. It was the complete *fin de siècle* outfit. I half expected to find Monsieur Renoir would be joining us.

She trod her way through the palace at Versailles, a tall, impressive, indeed imperious figure, who blended with the grand long windowed rooms as if she owned them. There were one or two guides taking groups of tourists round the magnificent building. She stopped near one of these and listened for a few moments, then banged the end of her parasol several times on the floor like a gavel. The crowd moved back as she made her way through to the guide. She told him the information he was dispensing was quite erroneous. He bowed in deference. Then Madame la Comtesse de Dampierre addressed the group in an unstoppable flow of words, and completed the tour to her satisfaction.

I was reminded of the scene many years later when I took my daughter Amanda, then aged twelve, to Rome for a birthday present. She was already well ahead of her years in Greek and Latin, and her passionate interest at the time was Greek and Roman mythology. We went round the Borghese Museum. To my surprise she politely interrupted the guide, and pointed out a mistake in what he had just said about the Bellini sculpture of Apollo and Daphne. Being Italian he started to argue, but her knowledge flowed over him like a waterfall from Parnassus. He then smiled, took her hand and asked her to be his assistant for the rest of the tour. Amanda accompanied him, prompting him from time to time, totally unselfconsciously. I followed in the crowd and hung on her words like the ignoramus I was in such matters, but I felt a rare pride in the whole proceedings.

After the Versailles outing, I felt it was time to go. I packed up, bade Elie and his mother goodbye and turned the car in the direction of Switzerland. All through the long drive I was intensely occupied with the problem of how I was going to make my money last out. The other side of Belfort I hit on a solution.

Herr Doktor Johann Hubermann was of stocky build, had large eyes behind horn-rimmed spectacles, a large mouth with large teeth and a large smile. His wife Gerda looked very similar except that small was the repetitive epithet. When I arrived in Rutikon, Zurich, their welcome was effusive. They rushed about and went in and out of doors for no apparent reason. I was reminded of the two figures which appear alternately in one of those wooden Swiss toy barometers which tell you if it's fine or wet. Inside their full-size house was a full-size cuckoo clock.

We sat at the dining-table covered with a damask white tablecloth and had a cup of coffee. Frau Hubermann had no English at all and Hubermann was a three per center. His syntax definitely needed brushing up. We conversed in a dog's dinner mixture of French, German and English.

Two facts emerged which changed the ground rules laid out in Hubermann's letter to me. One was that he was not a Doctor of Medicine, but of science and ran a small *Gummiwerke* or rubber factory in the little town; the other was that, in the interests of thoroughness, he had already engaged for some days another 'English' to help with the conversation. Two must be twice as good as one. The object of the exercise was that Hubermann should be fluent in English for his proposed export business visits to Britain and America.

Michael Bussey was a tall, thin and nervous young man, who had spent four years as a prisoner of war mostly in Poland and looked as if he was still suffering from malnutrition. He also spoke with a broad cockney accent. I foresaw difficulties but not immediately the fun to come. There was only one spare room and I was to be farmed out in a bedroom in a nearby house, though I would still come to Hubermann's for the benefit of his wife's kitchen. As I had a car, I gathered I should drive the Hubermanns about a lot of the time, except when we were not all going to the mountains mit the bicycles. 'Bicycles you will find here,' said the smiling Hubermann.

The first morning after a breakfast of half-cooked mushrooms on a small piece of rye bread, Bussey and I went down to the local Gasthof for a bottle of lager called Haldengut. The alternative Feldschlossen was even weaker. We were watched in silence, even suspicion by the other customers. Bussey spilt a small drop of beer on the table. Immediately the proprietor rushed up with a cloth, wiped the spot away, and polished the table vigorously with such sudden despatch that Bussey jumped.

'Bloody Krauts,' he said under his breath. 'The whole bloody place is like a prison camp.'

'What about the Hubermanns?' I asked. 'They seem harmless enough.'

'Listen mate,' said Bussey. 'They're a couple of mean sods. Tried to tell me Switzerland had a bad time in the war! You had the breakfast this morning?' I nodded. 'Well, that's about the biggest meal you'll get. Same every day. It's fucking awful.'

I drank some Haldengut and changed the subject.

'How have you been getting on with the old boy's English lessons?'

Bussey's face broke into a grin, exposing some broken teeth.

'I've been teaching 'im Cockney rhyming slang.'

I laughed and knew we were already entering into a conspiracy. There and then we worked out a few little linguistic tricks. The word 'bloody' was incessantly on Bussey's lips. We told Hubermann it was idiomatic for 'very'. He was soon declaring that the weather was bloody good. We had a lot of fun also with 'old boy' but that required a detailed explanation that the phrase had nothing to do with age. Bussey's 'grub' for food was checked in the dictionary by Hubermann and the answer puzzled him. We emphasized that we were really trying to give him the edge on his competitors by providing colloquialisms. This eventually paid off by his declaring his wife's offerings were 'bloody good grub'.

Our crowning achievement was about meeting in the mornings. At breakfast we instituted a serious little ceremony which we told Hubermann was a standard greeting in polite circles. We all stood seriously and shook hands. It was extremely difficult to keep a straight face as Hubermann said with a slight bow,

'Good morning, Mr. Thorn. Good morning Mr. Bussey. Wotcha cock!'

'Wotcha cock,' we replied and sat down to our mushrooms.

A short time later Hubermann asked me if I would take him in the Hillman to his brother's farm, half an hour into the mountains to pick up some food and goods. It was a dark and stormy night, and on the way we picked up two friends. We were five up in the car and as the journey up the hairpin-bends turned out to be nearly two hours, the old Hillman boiled over and sighed with a cloud of steam from sheer exhaustion when we reached our destination.

Hubermann and his friends loaded up the boot and the floor in front of the back seat with hams, large chunks of Gruyère, bacon, butter, eggs, garlic smelling salami and bottles of wine. We made our way down again without mishap, dropping off the friends with their shares on the way. When we had unloaded all these goodies back at Hubermann's with Bussey's help, he whispered to me, 'Well, we should get a bloody better breakfast tomorrow.'

But we were disappointed. The same mushrooms and bread appeared as usual.

I thought Bussey was going to explode.

'Where's all that bloody grub you brought back last night then?'

'Ah,' smiled Hubermann expansively. 'That I have into the refrigerator put for the winter.'

'I want a fuckin' egg,' said Bussey almost in tears. I thought of all the years he had suffered in Poland.

But Hubermann was adamant. Bussey packed the same day. I drove him to the station.

'Why are you going to stay?' he asked.

'I haven't enough cash to get home,' I said.

'Well good luck, mate,' he waved from the carriage window.

'Wotcha cock,' I said. The train disappeared down the line.

I still had another four weeks to stay with Hubermann. The only asset I had was my watercolours. I painted like mad all over the Zurcher Oberland and managed about twenty-five. I sold a dozen of these to a tourist shop in Rapperswill and recouped the necessary sum to be on my way. On my last night, lighting a cigarette at the table after the special treat of *fondu*, the little flat wooden match broke and landed on the table cloth. Hubermann slapped his large hand over it. But there was a millimetre diameter black-edged hole left behind. Frau Hubermann burst into tears, because the cloth was a wedding present from her mother. Hubermann danced about like a maniac. I offered to get the tiny hole invisibly repaired but this was met with a stream of words by both of them in their strange northern Swiss dialect. They retired to another room for a conference. I finished my cigarette and stubbed it out very carefully in the ashtray.

Hubermann returned and sat at the table opposite me. He pointed to the tiny hole.

'My wife wants a new tablecloth. You will have to buy it.'

'But it's ridiculous. This can easily be mended.'

'New tablecloth,' repeated Hubermann.

'I can't afford that,' I said. 'I've only just enough cash to get home.'

Hubermann sucked on his teeth loudly.

'*Ach so*,' he said. 'I will all your pictures instead take.'

I shook my head and used a well-known English phrase.

'Not bloody likely. You can have three and *I'll* choose them.'

'OK,' he said. 'You can pay me the rest when I to London come.'

And that's how it was left. I went the next morning. It seemed to be becoming a habit that I left everywhere I went under some sort of cloud.

When I reached Paris, I called on the Comtesse and Elie and asked his mother to choose two pictures as a gift from me. She was entranced. *'Charmantes, les petites aquarelles charmantes. Merci beaucoup,'* and then *'Bon voyage, Monsieur.'*

My next call was to Rolande. I telephoned her, and she told me she was just about to leave Paris to stay with her sister in Normandy. I went round to her flat and she came down with her baggage which I put in the car to take her to the Gare Saint Lazare. I then gave her the money owed to her for past services rendered. She was astounded. She flung her arms round my neck and gave me a long passionate kiss. *'Incroyable! Les Anglais, les Anglais,'* she laughed. *'Ils sont tous sympathiques.'* Then she put the notes swiftly into her handbag.

'As tu de Players?' she asked.

I gave her my last full packet and watched her totter down the platform in her high heels.

When I reached Boulogne the night before the car-ferry left the next morning, I filled up the tank with petrol and discovered I hadn't enough francs left to get a bed even in a simple pension.

I looked at the faithful old Hillman.

'I'll have to sleep with you tonight, old boy,' I muttered.

I found a suitable place to park. Then I saw a signpost. Le Touquet. What could I lose, I thought, I have to stay the night in the car anyway.

I had never been inside a casino but a boy at school had brought a roulette set one term, and I was familiar with the general principles. As I was in Gaul, I divided the remaining francs into three equal parts. Which were the lucky numbers? Number 2 the Schools, Number 18 Beaumont Street or 23 Craven Street? Eighteen and twenty-three went down. I put my last francs on number two. It came up at thirty-six to one.

I took the chips to the cashier, collected the money and drove to the Westminster Hotel which had just re-opened. I booked into a double bedroom with balcony, and ordered some pâté and a bottle of champagne in the room.

As I waited for the waiter to wheel in my simple supper I put my feet up on the bed and watched the grey white horses of the channel which stretched across to England. I felt it was a fitting conclusion to my first trip abroad.

13 Box Office

My Membership examination was in early January 1947. My caperings across France and Switzerland had provided a holiday and heady tonic, but the three and a half remaining months of 1946 demanded intensive study if I was going to turn in any sort of academic performance in this highly competitive examination. I got down to it with vigour and application but things were going on in my head, and indeed my body, which were insistent and compulsive.

I was still living at my father's expense doing the postgraduate courses at Hammersmith, the West End Hospital for Nervous Diseases, the Skin hospital in Lisle Street, Soho, and the Royal National Orthopaedic.

Two things happened which interrupted this austere programme. One was the character of Hubermann. The play I had promised myself had to be written. I shut myself up in Barkston Gardens and wrote the three acts of *Mit the Bicycles* in the same number of weeks. I went home with the script and read it to my father. He laughed all the way through, made a few additions and criticisms. My mother typed every word. With the help of Humphrey Perkins Gestetner we rolled off fifty copies, collated them on the long benches in the chemistry lab, and had them bound in Melton Mowbray with a printed cover by an old friend of my father's.

The reason I had so many copies done was because from past experience I had found it took about three months to get a reply about a script from a theatrical management. I worked out that with all the try-out theatres added in, if I were to submit them one by one it would take some ten years before the whole market had been explored. I therefore sent forty copies out simultaneously (keeping ten in reserve) on the first of January 1947. It seemed fair enough to me to let everyone have the same chance to snap up this masterpiece.

The second event which diverted me was that I met Thelma who was doing a beautician's training course at Maria Hornes in Davies Street. She was a very glamorous creature. My resolve to marry a French girl – all of whom I thought, erroneously, would be as accommodating and expert as Rolande – disappeared. I fell in love overnight with Thelma, whose home was in Chippenham.

I sat the Membership papers in a building in Queen Square.

There was an enormous entry of five hundred candidates, some trying for the tenth time. I learnt only twenty-five or so would be passed. I got through to the final viva reached by about fifty candidates.

On 15 January two letters arrived at Barkston Gardens. One told me I had just failed the Membership by a narrow margin but I was urged to sit the next examination in June. The other letter contained a contract for *Mit the Bicycles* from Jack de Leon who ran the 'Q' Theatre. If I accepted, the advance on royalties would be £100. I got straight on the phone home with the bad news and the good news. Father accepted the bad stoically and offered no criticisms. I could tell from his voice he was very excited about the good.

'Get Ted Eveleigh to vet the contract,' he said, 'And get an agent.' Ted, by then a Junior Barrister in Armstrong-Jones's chambers, very kindly obliged *gratis*. I read down the list of play agents in the *Author's Yearbook*. The only name I knew was Vosper. I rang Margery and asked her if she was related to Frank Vosper, the author of *Love from a Stranger*, the film of which I had seen.

'Yes,' she said. 'Frank was my late brother.' I told her about Jack de Leon's offer, and went down to her office in Shaftesbury Avenue. As with the several plays she subsequently handled for me she made the same disconcerting remark. 'What a joke!'

She rang Jack de Leon, made a few minor adjustments to the contract and told me to sign it. The title was altered to *Mountain Air* and we went into rehearsal in early April, after Hedley Briggs the producer had cut at least forty-five minutes out of the overlong script. Martin Miller played Hubermann – a positive facsimile – and Geoffrey Sumner tailored Michael Bussey into a demobbed Wing Commander with great effect. Mary Martlew, and Avice Landone were also in the cast.

In the meantime I heard from Justin Power that he had got *The Man in the Market Place*, of which he was co-author, accepted for a Holy Week run by the Northampton Repertory Theatre, the play being billed as a 'Modern Passion Play'. We made up our differences to some degree and the play had a good reception in March.

On the strength of all this intoxicating stuff, I proposed to Thelma. When I relayed this intelligence to my father and told him I was going to get married, he asked astutely, 'What on? Hadn't you better get a job? There's no more from this end.'

Malcolm Sargent accompanied by a beautiful companion and my parents came to the first night of *Mountain Air* at 'Q'. Malcolm and my father led the laughter, and set the tone for the whole audience. Later in the week the Daniel Meyer Company bought the play for the Comedy Theatre. In the meantime I sent for my other scripts back and collected a series of vituperative letters from many managements telling me I just could not send out more than one script at a time. I also was forwarded a reader's report covered in ringed coffee-cup stains which said the play was not a play at all, would never get produced and could never possibly reach the West End.

Having met Alex Boyd, the accountant of Associated British Pictures for whom my schoolfriend John Redway was casting director, Alex offered me his flat in Linden Gardens, Notting Hill Gate, rent free while he went to America for six months. With £30 to my credit in the bank, Thelma and I were married on 7 May in Kensington Parish Church and Roger Frisby was my best man. We went to Portmeirion in North Wales for our honeymoon, Nap and Joan de Rouet putting a case of vintage Bollinger in our car boot as a wedding present. Each night I fired a cork down the little cliff into the sea. When we returned, I started a job as assistant to a GP in Greenford, a Doctor Murray. Life seemed intensely exciting. I planned no further attempts at the Membership.

Dr. Murray was a keen efficient doctor whose practice was growing. That is why he needed an assistant. His home, surgery, and garage were in Greenford Road. His wife did the accounts. It was a year before the National Health Service started and the old Panel system was operating very well. The patients were mixed working and middle class, the latter being private patients. I was paid seven pounds ten a week and provided my own car, petrol and lunch. I was pleased to learn Murray did all the night calls himself, so that after evening surgery I sped back to the flat in Linden Gardens to sample Thelma's cooking experiments. Her hands were too well manicured to peel potatoes, so I insisted we used a ghastly preparation called 'Pom', the forerunner of 'Smash'. But we in fact ate out a lot, for a few shillings at local snack bars.

All the walls of Alex Boyd's flat were covered to ceiling height with signed photographs of the stars, most of whom I was later to examine. We made love with abandon under this plethora of celluloid glamour, male and female.

The day before I officially started my six-months contract 'with view', Murray explained that visits were done on a cash basis. He gave me a street map of his territory and I made notes on it about the charges while he drove me round.

'These are all five-shilling touches,' he would say of a particular street. 'Both sides. Except the corner house there which is seven and six. I'll do the ten bob ones myself.'

I soon found that money for the rent, the rates, the gas, the electricity were saved in different pots in various parts of the houses. The doctor's cut usually had pride of place in the centre of the mantel-piece. I found the system fair and effective and no one complained or seemed to be yearning for the seemingly free bonanza which Bevan was promising them. The only drawback was that by the end of a visiting round all my pockets were full of coppers and other small coins which weighed me down and rattled as I walked, like a rag and bone man after a good day. I arrived back at Murray's with the loot and emptied it in a huge heap on the dining-table where Mrs. Murray presided at the seat of custom. She quickly made neat piles of coins with the practical hands of a bank clerk, checked my visiting list and gave me a cup of coffee and a biscuit. Only once was I a penny short. After two recounts I found the coin in one of my trouser turnups. Panic was averted and honour satisfied.

In Linden Gardens I started writing a new play, this time a thriller, about a crazed lorry driver who bullied his girlfriend and terrorized his family and ran a 'Good Pull-up for Car Men' on a lonely stretch of Watling Street which runs up the Edgware Road to Holyhead. I called it *A5*, repeated the fifty copy procedure and sent it out.

This time the response was even quicker than for *Mountain Air*. Thelma and I had just returned to the flat from a meal of fish and chips, to find the phone ringing. It was Marjorie Hawtrey who ran the Embassy Theatre, Swiss Cottage. She was bubbling with enthusiasm: they wanted to do it. Would we like to join them there and then at the Savoy Grill so that I could meet the producer, Michael Macowan, who had just successfully launched one of Priestley's plays. Repeating the Eveleigh-Brandt formula we went straight down in a taxi, and carried out what amounted to a casting meeting at the table. We demolished roast duck, green peas and champagne.

The cast included Elwyn Brook Jones, Alfie Bass, Sydney Taffler and Mary Horn. The title was again changed for the better to *Headlights on A5* and the play was put on for four weeks in the summer. The reviews were mixed. It was really a kitchen-sink drama but unfortunately ten years too early for the trend, so it did not transfer to the West End.

The young film director Lewis Gilbert tried to get the play filmed but missed by a hair's breadth.

By the autumn I was in a breathless state of anticipation about *Mountain Air*, but the play running at the Comedy, *The Crime of Margaret Foley*, refused to come off until December. However, my bank balance was looking a little more healthy.

I was dithering as to whether to renew my contract with Murray when again Ted Eveleigh came into my life and made a suggestion which I followed. He asked me if I had ever thought of doing medico-legal reports and did I mind going into Court to give evidence? I told him of my court martial experience at Bournemouth and he warned me that the High Court was quite a different matter. After very little hesitation, the fee of three guineas per report was irresistible. I signed off with Murray, Alex Boyd returned from America, and Thelma and I moved into a basement furnished flat in Gloucester Gate, Regent's Park. We made some more love, this time to the faint sounds of roaring lions at the zoo.

To Ted I shall always be eternally indebted for launching me on my medico-legal career, and hence my insurance practice.

My first case came from E. R. Phillips of Bingham and Co., Solicitors, acting on instructions from Ken Douglass of the Paladin. I still get cases from these two sources. I found the practice ideal, for it left my evenings and weekends free for writing. Appearances in the witness-box were terrifying at first but with my dramatic interests, the sheer theatre of the court-room became a double pleasure.

At this early stage I was lucky to meet Sir Hugh Griffiths who was a master of the craft of being an expert medical witness. He gave me a very useful tip which I have tried to follow. After a consultation together he said. 'Look Thorn, the only way to write a sound reliable report devoid of any bias is to examine the patient, dictate your opinion and then read your instructing letter to see whether you are acting for the Plaintiff or the Defendant. That's the way to build your reputation. Good luck to you.'

By the beginning of 1948 we were able to move from Regent's Park to a leasehold flat in Weymouth Street in the centre of the medical area where I could both live and practise. I did not join the new National Health Service. The idea of doctors getting a single capitation fee for each patient on his list regardless of the number of times seen, and the fact that a doctor received the same reward whether he was conscientious, good, bad or indifferent seemed to fly in the face of human nature. The running of the whole thing by a largely lay bureaucratic controlling body was totally offputting. The scheme was also based on Health Centres, of which there was only one in existence when it started. Though agreeing with the idealistic principles involved, I predicted the NHS would break down financially. But it took forty-five years longer than I anticipated to reach its present chaotic state.

The first night of *Mountain Air* at the Comedy was in January 1948. It had good reviews, and without a star name in the cast ran for nearly eight months. It then went on two provincial tours, was performed on radio and TV, was published by Samuel French and still all these years later brings in a tiny income.

Jack de Leon installed a laughter machine outside the theatre, which relayed the audience reaction on a giant-sized thermometer, the indicator shooting up and down with each gust of mirth.

During the run of the play I had a phone-call from Hubermann. He was in London on his first sales trip for the *Gummiwerke*. Thelma had the chance to him hospitality offer. True to form he collected for the purchase of a new tablecloth from me the money and produced a gift for Thelma, which he made quite a big production number out of. It was a single, admittedly large, bar of Toblerone. On the strength of this we took him out to dinner to the Comedy Restaurant opposite the theatre.

I must admit to a certain satisfaction, while we ate, at hearing the laughter from across the street which his stage Doppelganger, Martin Miller, was provoking. Which brings us nearly back to where we came in.

My practice developed not only because of its instigation by Ted but also because of Ronnie Armstrong-Jones, who was a Silk doing the same litigation work and whom we met with Ted at an insurance company's Claims Department annual dance. Afterwards we went along to Rico's Casanova and Don Juan Club which had just opened.

Thelma and I became very friendly with Ronnie Armstrong-Jones and his actress wife Carol Coombe. At one time the friendship got too hectic and indeed far too expensive for me to keep up with. Eventually I had to stoop to ruses to counter the flood of invitations. These invariably arrived somewhat late at night. I can hear now that querulous if not tremulous voice on the bedside phone.

'Hello. . .o . . . my dear fellow. Here we are . . . Carol and I . . . at the Casanova . . . Come on down and join us . . . What? In bed? But it's only eleven-thirty . . . positively disgusting . . . What? . . . Well, put on your clothes my dear fellow . . . Champers cocktails all lined up . . . look forward to seeing you . . .' And the message would end with a click. We usually tottered home again about four-thirty and the astounding thing was that after such a late night I sometimes found myself in the witness box in the High Court by ten-thirty, feeling decidedly slow if not slightly hesitant in my answers to Ronnie's searching questions of an expert witness. Though at least twenty years older, he seemed as bright as paint and devastatingly alert, which only shows what training and practice will accomplish.

At one point I became so exhausted that, wishing to avoid a weekend session at Addison Road where they held frequent parties, Thelma and I escaped to Paris having told only one person 'in the strictest confidence' where we were. On the Saturday morning we were just leisurely enjoying our coffee and croissants in our room at the Napoleon when the phone rang and the familiar voice bleated from the other end of the line.

'Hello, Ronnie . . . Tracked you down my dear fellow . . . Here we are at the Ritz bar . . . Come on, Carol and I are both waiting for you . . . Champers cocktails all laid on . . . see you in half an hour.' And that was the end of the quiet weekend.

We duly had the drinks and I was delighted that I was not going to have to share the cost of the lunch at the Ritz. But I needn't have worried. Ronnie walked us miles to 'a terribly fashionable bistro' on the left bank, 'And cheap my dears – fantastic.'

Ronnie's magnanimity was irresistible. When he announced, after we had eaten, that he was going to buy Carol and Thelma a bottle of scent each, we traipsed back to the Passy area: 'Never trust these French cab-drivers, old boy.' Inside a chic *parfumerie* not far from the George V, Ronnie had the two sales-ladies proffer the girls every test bottle in the shop. The final purchase were two little handbag sprays. Ronnie was undaunted by the voluble Gallic observations and gestures as we trooped out of the establishment.

But Ronnie had the ineffable charm of gaiety and *joie de vivre* which enlivened any gathering and our life would have been deficient in many respects had we not enjoyed his friendship. He had a tendency towards practical jokes which only rarely fell flat. I remember particularly one evening at the Caprice. In the bar he sported a bow tie which bore little jewels. These unaccountably flashed intermittently. Being a master of production he operated the bulb in his pocket for an occasional split-second so that one was not quite sure if one had really seen the sudden sparkle or not. Combined with a dead-pan expression the joke was surprisingly effective. Later Ronnie excused himself before the hors d'oeuvres and returned for the entrée fully bearded. It is a tribute to the skill of Mario as a famous restaurateur that, while we were in hysterics, he wore as impassive an expression as Ronnie. He then removed the hairy encumbrance as he found that asparagus proved an impossible task.

Our friendship was not in any way diminished by the episode which I like to call 'The story of the three doctors and the four cigars'.

One winter Saturday night Ronnie rang me. To my surprise it was not an invitation to a night-club. I detected a note of anxiety which crystallized into a plea for me to drop everything and come down to his mother-in-law's flat in Cheyne Walk where she had been stricken by an attack of abdominal pain of some severity. 'It's her gall-bladder, old boy. Bring some morphine. Carol is beside herself, and the old girl refuses to go to the hospital.'

I responded with alacrity and carrying my emergency bag – black leather, gold initials – at the ready I entered the lift of the block of flats down by the river. Just as I was closing the gates of the lift, someone else entered carrying a bag – black leather, gold initials.

'I'm going to the fourth floor,' I said.

'So am I,' was the reply.

As I pushed the button, we eyed each other covertly. But it was no real surprise that we arrived outside the door of the same flat. I rang the bell. Ronnie appeared and let us in, and with consummate ease introduced us doctor to doctor as though we were two contestants in some sort of fight. Carol appeared and ushered us into her mother's bedroom.

Lady Coombe was lying in bed with a rapturous expression on her face. A very senior surgeon was palpating her abdomen, his eyes closed in concentration. Eventually he moved away from the bed and treated the two newcomers to a wintry smile. He washed his hands and then left the room.

My companion of the lift felt the lady's abdomen, and somewhat superfluously I followed suit. Lady Coombe seemed to have lost any pain from which she had recently suffered, and smiled at us benevolently as we left the room.

The surgeon was handing a piece of notepaper to Carol.

'Give her this if she wakes in the night. Call me in the morning if you're worried. Is there somewhere we can talk?'

Ronnie showed us into a small salon.

'My diagnosis is –'

'Spastic Colon,' I said.

'Spastic Colon,' repeated my lift chum.

'Precisely,' said the surgeon. 'Goodnight gentlemen.'

We went out into the hall. Ronnie ushered us to the flat door. As I was about to follow the other two, a grip on my arm restrained me. As the door shut Ronnie burst into effusive apologies.

'Ronnie, my dear friend,' he said. 'I am so sorry about those other two. When the old dear was all doubled up I panicked, I'm afraid. You know, started ringing everybody, but I do assure you, the only opinion I value is yours. What's your diagnosis?'

'Too many doctors upset the patient.' I smiled. 'No, we're all agreed. She'll be quite OK.'

'What a relief,' said Carol.

'Splendid, splendid, my dear fellow. How about a glass of champers?'

'Thank you,' I said.

Ronnie began opening a bottle.

'I can't begin to tell you how I appreciate your turning out at night like this. I shall expect a whacking great fee from you.'

'I wouldn't dream of sending a bill,' I said, and swallowed the proferred Moët. 'I don't mind turning out at night for a patient, it's the late night-club summons that shatters me.'

Ronnie roared with laughter. 'Point taken,' he said.

'But you'll have to have something,' said Carol. 'Ronnie, what about some cigars?'

'Do you smoke cigars?' he asked.

'Yes, sometimes,' I replied.

'I told you he did,' said Carol. 'Shall I get them?'

'I'll send you some round tomorrow,' cut in Ronnie.

And he was as good as his word. When I opened the package I discovered one of those slipover cardboard cartons which usually contain five half Coronas. This one had four – and one empty space.

Escape from people at times and from giving gratuitous medical advice and treatment at others are features of life in general and medical practice in particular.

These were combined in one early holiday in the South of France. After a punishing drive through the heat of Provence Thelma and I arrived at one of our favourite small hotels with its own private beach and two star Michelin food. We parked the car in a slot under the rattan sun awning. The azure blue of the sea, the cloudless sky, and the sawing of the *cigalles* seemed a haven of peace and quiet. We drank it all in without speaking.

Suddenly there was the sound of a car door slam followed by a long wail of pain. I got out and ran across the car park. An excited French family were clustered round *Grandpère* who had pinched his thumb. I declared my credentials and asked to look at the injury. The thumb-nail was partially avulsed and bleeding. Nothing serious but painful enough. I applied a simple dressing, gave the old boy some Codis tablets, and dispensed reassurance in Tomblingian French.

That evening on the terrace we were sipping our first Pastis when *Grandpère* appeared and sat some tables away. His thumb and whole hand were wrapped in voluminous bandages and his arm was in a sling.

'You see that,' I said to Thelma. 'The only effect will be to make his arm and hand quite stiff!'

The old man's daughter came over to us and poured out effusive thanks for my earlier attentions.

'But you will understand, Monsieur, we thought he should see a proper French doctor.'

'I understand perfectly,' I said, a little nettled. 'But see he moves his arm or it will seize up very quickly at his age.'

'Oh, no,' she said. 'He has been ordered to keep it absolutely still.'

I tried to give an imitation of a French shrug copied from the workmen on the quayside of Boulogne.

'Perhaps Madame will accept this gift.'

The woman put a box of chocolates in Thelma's hand and went away. In the bedroom later, Thelma opened the box. It was full of pieces of sweaty marzipan.

'I don't like marzipan,' said Thelma biting into one of them. 'And they're quite stale,' she added making a face. 'How dare they?'

I took the box into the bathroom and dropped it into the waste bin.

'Come on darling,' I said, 'we're not going to let a little tired marzipan spoil our holiday.'

We got into bed and were just going off to sleep when there came loud laughter from the next room.

'I know that laugh!' I exclaimed. 'That's Sillisand.'

'Who?'

'A Doctor Sillisand and if he's staying here we shan't have a minute to ourselves. Terrible bore.'

As if to prove my assertion a man in swimming trunks climbed on to our balcony.

'Coooee!' he called heartily. 'Thought it was you I saw, Thorn. Come on out for a swim in the moonlight.'

It was Sillisand all right. We declined the offer. He told us he'd be at the the hotel for a fortnight.

'So will we,' I said foolishly.

'Whacko. Lots of fun. See you.'

We heard him laughing all the way down to the water's edge.

'We shall have to move,' I said.

'What? From the hotel?' asked Thelma.

'Unless you want to be submerged in endless old jokes and involved in indefatigable physical activity. I tell you, I know Sillisand. Now go to sleep. We'll pack up early, be off, and find somewhere else.'

Thelma turned over and used a very unladylike word.

'Bugger,' she said.

To which there was no suitable reply.

We extricated ourselves from our reservation and were just putting the cases back in the car the next morning when Sillisand appeared still in his swimming trunks. It occurred to me that he might have been swimming all night.

'Hello hello hello,' he greeted us. 'What's all this then?'

'I, er, I'm afraid we've got to go back home,' I said. 'Very urgent case.'

'What about your partner?'

'Don't have one.'

'Should have. I've got two. Pity. I was looking forward to our getting together a whole lot,' he said eyeing Thelma.

'So were we,' she replied rapidly putting on her sun glasses.

'Well, bon voyage. Jolly bad luck. 'Bye for now.'

He trotted away into the hotel.

With quite a bit of luck we found a place about five miles along the coast. Again we were just settling down to our *apéritif* when Thelma looked startled.

'What's the matter?' I asked.

'Listen!'

I listened. The laugh was unmistakable.

'My God,' I said. 'We'd better hide.'

But we were too late. Sillisand had spotted us. For the first time the perpetual smile left his face.

'Just came along here for a drink,' he said. 'I thought you had an urgent case.'

'Snuffed before I could get there,' I replied.

He got the message at last and went off to join his party. He was soon laughing again.

On our way home, believe it or not, somewhere near Lyon's, as we were filling up with petrol, his car drew up for the same reason.

We each raised our hands briefly in a feeble greeting but there was no conversation and certainly no laughter.

14 'Roll 'Em'

For the next few years which took me out of the forties and into the fifties I settled down in Weymouth Street to my practice, my writing and to married life. The last produced two daughters, Amanda in 1950, and Vanessa in 1952, who have both remained a joy, comfort and delight to the present day. They have married stalwart chaps, each named Richard and for confusion's sake, each refusing to be called Dick. One lives in San Francisco, and one in Dulwich, which is not nearly as dull as it sounds. Vanessa has produced two daughters Sarah and Claire, and Amanda a son, Jonathan.

During the fifties I was steadily gaining an expertise in dealing with claims. These spanned the whole spectrum of medical conditions. People, I discovered, were very litigious. Amongst the main cases of serious head injuries and limb fractures, there were some bizarre diversions. An early one was the woman who sued a hotel in Brighton for being served maggots in green pea soup. The dish was refused and a second one provided – containing an even larger ration of the offending creatures. This was too much. She and her husband left the hotel in high dudgeon and when they got home to London the wife developed abdominal pain and anorexia. She was processed through a number of investigations like Barium meals, and blood tests by her doctor. By the time I saw her for the insurers of the hotel, a year later, she claimed she had never felt well since the incident and could not eat a thing. As she was over twelve stone in weight this statement seemed at best an exaggeration. In court I pointed out that cooked maggots were harmless and in any event were first-class protein as opposed to the second class of the green peas. Damages for psychological shock were awarded, but the sum was a good deal less than the amount hoped for.

There were other cases on the food front in amongst the hairdressing burns, the facial scars, the neck whip-lashes, the slipped discs and the loss of fingers and toes. The mouse is an ubiquitous rodent which turns up in various disguises. One of them appeared as a strawberry in the jam served at a famous London hotel. The guest was an old dear who came up to town each year from Cheltenham before Christmas to buy her presents and entertain her aged cronies. She adored strawberry jam but recoiled in horror as she bit through the largest of the fruit. The hotel wisely settled the claim without a fight.

There was another macabre instance when a customer purchased some bottled plums to discover half a human index finger at the bottom of the jar. The strange thing was that after extensive investigation the owner of the digit was never tracked down in farm, factory, warehouse or shop.

There is of course the celebrated case of the man who introduced a dead cockroach, from an empty matchbox carried in his pocket, on to his plate in a restaurant in London. He obtained damages, bided his time and eighteen months later repeated the coup in Birmingham. The third attempt in Edinburgh might also have succeeded had not a member of the same insurance company's claims department been transferred to Scotland – the name of the claimant rang a bell. He got several years for fraud.

Of course these affairs are not so funny when one is on the receiving end. I had to go with Lippy Kessel to East Anglia to deal with the claim of an actress who was playing *The Wife of Bath* and had torn a calf muscle leaping repeatedly out of the location bed.

Zeffirelli, the director, invited us to dinner and I was sitting next to him. He asked me it I would like an English translation of the Italian script of *The Canterbury Tales,* but the irony of the question was lost on me, as I swallowed a dead wasp which I had not seen in the Bloody Mary I was drinking.

One Christmas dinner – which Thelma always served on Christmas Eve – Amanda, then about seven, stopped masticating her mouthful of turkey and gave a cry of distaste as her face froze in horror.

'Whatever's the matter, Amanda?' I asked. Moving her lips as little as possible and keeping her mouth half open, she mumbled tearfully,

'There's a beetle . . .'

Indeed something black was protruding from her lips amidst the dark red of the cranberry sauce.

'It's just a dark piece of cranberry skin,' I reassured her.

'It's a beetle,' she wailed.

'Then spit it out.'

'You'll do no such thing,' said her mother peering at the child slightly short-sightedly. 'Eat it up!'

After a brief hesitation, Amanda obeyed the word of authority with commendable fortitude. The crisis over, I was about to savour my first mouthful of the meal when I saw on my fork the unmistakable head and antennae of a member of the Coleoptera, the common black beetle *Broscus cephalotes.*

'My God,' I exclaimed. 'She's right. It *is* a beetle.' Thelma rose to her feet in fury. 'That's it!' she said. 'The whole meal's ruined. And it's your fault,' she glared at me accusingly. 'You bought the cranberry sauce. I shall never cook another Christmas dinner again,' and steamed out of the room.

The only person who seemed to enjoy the affair was Vanessa who was laughing uncontrollably at Amanda's discomfiture. I think this was because of an earlier crisis when Vanessa had got her foot stuck between the spokes of a tricycle wheel. I tried to release her but she shouted out painfully.

'Keep still,' I said. 'I shall have to cut it off,' meaning of course her sandal. Amanda in glee ran off to tell Mummy. 'Come and watch. Daddy's going to cut Vanessa's foot off.'

When we moved to Lister House in Wimpole Street I acquired with the flat a new piece of medical equipment invaluable in my special field. It was an ornate but sturdy stone balcony on to which one could walk from french windows. This allowed me to observe unseen patients after they had left, as they emerged into the street and went on their way after their quest for compensation. It is illuminating to see a man who had been unable to get across the consulting room, without a marked limp, stride down the steps of the building and walk briskly away. This valuable clinical sign inclines me not to disbelieve the hoary old medico-legal story of the claimant in court seeking compensation for an injury to his shoulder. When requested by the judge to show how far he could raise his arm, he brought it up painfully to the horizontal. When asked how far he could raise it before his accident, he shot his hand up unguardedly well above his head, and secured a quick dismissal of his case.

In a lecture I gave called 'Claims, Hysteria, and Malingering' to the Insurance Institute of London, which later published it in their journal, I gave some other instances:

A malingerer tends to over-impress the examiner with the severity of his pain or tenderness. At the same time, by an exaggerated show of endeavour, he seeks to demonstrate how hard he is trying and what a genuine chap he is. He cries out in pain when attempting to move his painful back; he grunts and puffs and blows, and contorts his whole body. A truly painful back makes the patient avoid all unnecessary movement.

The malingerer rarely complains of loss of sensation in an injured part as does the true hysteric. Even the duller witted realize that a sharp pin is too available a weapon to show up their counterfeit. The very tough may try it, but clenching of the hands and jaws and sweating give the game away under this torture.

The malingerer often loses his signs when he thinks he is unobserved or is off his guard. The same hand which can only produce a feeble grip during the examination shakes the examiner's warmly when the imposter says goodbye, imagining he has come safely through his ordeal with all his colours of deception flying. The malingerer who has lost his voice can cough quite loudly, although in each case the larynx is used. As is said in one of Fontaine's fables, 'The Cock and the Fox', it is a double pleasure to deceive the deceiver. I remember one case where a man had a frightful limp and stiff leg and had to be literally helped across the consulting room. He wore an abominable purple and yellow large check sports jacket. About an hour and a half later, driving down Baker Street, I noticed a similarly attired figure sprinting hard and leaping on to a bus. There could not have been two jackets like that. As it turned out in court, there were not.

A colleague who went to examine an ostensibly bed-ridden patient at her home, mistook the day of the appointment and arrived to carry out his examination a day early. He was admitted by a relative and was kept waiting for some time but within earshot of much scuffling in the bedroom. When at last he went up to see the good lady he found that in her hurry to prepare for her pathetic bed-ridden state, she had slipped up on a small but significant detail. She was lying in bed in her night-dress but was still wearing her hat.

Such is the prevalence of claims for personal damages and their rewards, that after one examination of a burly warehouse-man, with a genuine injury and for whose union I had examined him, he praised me for the thoroughness of my examination and as he left he tipped me half-a-crown for my efforts.

Prevention is of course cheaper than cure. A surgeon colleague once told me that as he turned a corner sharply in his car, a pedestrian stepped off the pavement. Fortunately, my friend managed to pull up an inch from his victim. Expecting the usual tirade of abuse, he was somewhat taken aback by the remark, 'Why did you stop, Guv'nor? I needed that money.'

Dealing with claims in the film industry presents an entirely different problem. The artiste who is ill or injured is not the claimant. It is the production company who is asking the insurers of the picture to indemnify them for loss of shooting time, with astronomical costs mounting each day. All the other stars and artistes, the film crew, technicians, who remain on full pay until the disabled actor or actress is fit enough to shoot once more, have to be paid, not to mention studio and location rent. If the condition is very serious, re-casting and starting all over again becomes a possibility or even abandonment of the film might be considered.

The financial pressures can be enormous and often at the sharp end of all this is the insurance doctor who has to give a prognosis. The pressures put on him derive from all sides – the film company, the insurers and the artiste himself – to give the answer which is correct and if possible makes everyone happier.

There are undercurrents of a power struggle which are not always immediately perceived. Suppressed panic and the fear of financial disaster is always in the air, and time is of the essence. The bells ring and off one has to go immediately to a stricken location. Lavish VIP travel and hospitality is invariably offered. Persuasion towards a certain medical conclusion is lobbied from all sides, and this often includes conflicting opinions from the star's own medical advisers and other medical men who are brought into the act from various sources. The insurance doctor's integrity has to remain paramount and his nerve towards this end must remain unshakable and authoritative. Not an easy assignment as I have often found out. One's fees are certainly earned.

Sometimes the producer tries one on if he has decided, say two weeks after shooting begins, he is not happy with his director or cast and seeks a medical reason to make a change, and thereby recover insurance costs which he would otherwise have to finance himself. The suggestion that someone is showing signs of mental instability or is on drugs has to be tested clinically with totally unbiased acumen. I was once subjected by a producer to a long quasi-medical diagnosis of a particular director's problem even before I had seen the patient. The treatment advised was to give the director a long rest to get over his obvious nervous breakdown. I eventually stopped this softening up process by asking the producer where he had qualified medically. The director was quite fit apart from a head cold. There were no medical grounds for his removal and he completed the picture successfully without further trouble.

At other times things are easy. I flew to Limerick for *The Last Remake of Beau Geste*. The film and whole unit were at a total standstill. A very young local doctor had pronounced that Marty Feldman the director had smallpox. I blame the doctor not at all. It is sometimes a difficult diagnosis in the early stages. By the time I got there a tell-tale pathognomonic lesion in the centre of the soft palate confirmed the presence of chickenpox and everyone heaved a sigh of relief.

Though I have supreme admiration for American medicine and the overwhelming contribution of the United States to research, the clinical approach is weighted differently from the British one. The tendency often seems in most cases to run every conceivable laboratory and ancillary test, see what the results throw up and then look at the patient. This is an expensive, time-consuming way of doing things. On the other hand it is exhaustively thorough. I suppose every doctor's nightmare is that he should miss something.

During one film being made in Britain, Marlon Brando was admitted to the private wing of a London teaching hospital. A diagnosis was reached and appropriate treatment proposed. But before this was carried out Marlon insisted on one of his own personal physicians flying over from Los Angeles to check things out.

The senior surgeon and the West End GP engaged by the production company had so far been in charge. I was called in to hold a watching brief for the insurers. The three of us waited for the great man's arrival. All reasonable tests had been done but from experience of the film world I warned my two colleagues that the American physician would certainly demand many more.

Dr. Borsito arrived. He was the perfect type-cast for the

Hollywood doctor of that era – in his fifties, greying crew cut hair, a sharp dark suit, steel rimmed spectacles and of serious mien. He shook hands with us solemnly.

'Gentlemen, I guess I should first let Marlon know I'm here. Then we can evaluate the problem afterwards. He's in . . .?'

The GP indicated the door to the private ward. The three of us followed Borsito and stood behind him at the end of the bed like students.

'Marlon,' announced his physician. 'I am here.'

'Hi,' said Marlon.

'You therefore have nothing more to worry about.' Borsito waved his hand towards us, all complete strangers to him. 'And let me tell you, Marlon, you are also under the care of three of the finest doctors in Europe. Now you relax, Marlon, while we discuss your little problem.'

'Great,' said Marlon and we all trooped out again.

The GP produced all the blood tests, X-rays, IVP, Barium Enema and other investigations for Borsito to study which he did diligently. The surgeon was looking at his watch.

'Well,' said Borsito, 'I think we should have electrolytes, full liver profile and an ECG.'

'I'll get all those done,' said the GP and the meeting broke up.

By the time the tests were complete, and all proved normal, Marlon made a rapid and complete recovery and was back on the set in three days. I suppose you could say it was game, set and match to the Americans.

The German approach to orthopaedics is again different from ours.

During the filming of one of the Bond pictures, *On Her Majesty's Secret Service*, Ilsa Steppat tripped over a telephone cord in her own flat in West Berlin and fractured the shaft of her left humerus. This is a bone which usually heals very quickly. A simple collar and cuff sling for a few weeks followed by gentle exercises is all the treatment required. The film situation with Ilsa Steppat, whom I had examined before the film in London, was that she had done a few days' shooting at the beginning and was required for two more days on location in Portugal, at the end. The principal shots were of her in the rear of a car firing a revolver in her right hand. There seemed little problem, since skilful photography could disguise her left arm even if it were in a sling. But the successful James Bond film company had not taken into account Herr Professor Domrich who described himself as a War Surgeon and into whose authoritarian hands Ilsa Steppat had come. My telephone rang. The call was from Richard Youens of Graham

Miller & Co., Assessors for the Fireman's Fund.

'We have learnt,' I was told, 'that the German surgeon looking after Ilsa has put her in a bed in a private hospital, her arm is in a complicated splint, and he says she will not be fit for shooting until well after she is needed on location. We've got to have her on location because she's in a whole lot of the beginning of the picture. This means a big claim. Check it all out, Ronnie, will you? Go to Berlin and keep us informed.'

Richard rang off.

The first thing to do was to speak to Domrich and arrange a consultation. The Assessors supplied me with his address and number. After four attempts by my secretary, which took a whole day, I finally got hold of him. He did not speak English, so we conversed through an interpreter at the other end.

I learnt that the patient's arm was in an 'aeroplane' (abduction) splint. Traction applied through a pin inserted in the elbow had just been removed. This was a method we had given up in Britain for many years.

'She's in bed and will not be fit to film for a long time,' said Domrich through the interpreter.

'Tell the Professor,' I said, 'the insurers of the film wish me to come over and see her.'

'There's no need,' was the quick reply. 'Professor Domrich has given his opinion.'

'But I still have to make a report.'

'Quite unnecessary.'

'Tell Professor Domrich,' I said, 'it is a usual routine matter for the insurance. She is needed for shooting again very soon.'

'Impossible! Goodbye,' was the reply and the line went dead. I got another call through almost immediately.

'Professor Domrich,' I began.

'Professor Domrich does not need any English doctor to tell him how to treat one of his own patients,' cut in the interpreter.

'I'm not questioning his treatment [though of course I was], I merely wish to examine Miss Steppat and make a report for the insurance company. I will examine her only in the Professor's presence. I could be in Berlin tomorrow.'

'Tomorrow he is not available.'

'Then the day after?'

There was a long pause.

'He will see you at the Martin Luther Krankenhaus on Saturday at 10.00 a.m.'

'Thank you,' I said. 'I shall be there.'

Obviously things were going to be very tricky and difficult. But in fact far more than I imagined.

I flew to Berlin the night before the consultation, stayed at the

Kempinski and at 9.50 on the Saturday morning presented myself at the hospital. It was an impressive private clinic. I approached the reception desk.

'My name is Doctor Thorn. I have a consultation with Herr Professor Domrich to see Miss Ilsa Steppat at ten o'clock,' I said.

'Ya,' was the reply from the Clerk. 'I have a message for you from the Herr Professor. He has been called away for two days and will not be able to see you.'

'That's very unfortunate,' I said. 'Then perhaps I can see Miss Steppat and speak to Professor Domrich on the phone afterwards?'

'That is not allowed,' I was told.

'But I came from London last night and can't hang about here for two days.'

The clerk's head shook sadly.

'*Verboten.*'

'Now look here, this is ridiculous. Perhaps I could see the patient with the Herr Professor's assistant?'

'He is very busy.'

'But he *is* in the clinic?'

'Er . . .'

'Then will you please get him? This examination has to be carried out. I shall wait as long as is necessary.'

'But I have said, he is . . .'

I then raised my voice in what I imagined to be that of a German officer. '*Besorgen sie sich. Jetzt!*' and banged my case on the desk. There was a flicker of hesitation and then, '*Ya, Herr Doktor,*' said the clerk.

I was kept waiting nearly an hour and then a young good looking doctor appeared carrying a file of notes and an X-ray envelope. Another interpreter materialized, but he turned out not to be necessary as the doctor in due course spoke to me in fluent English. He conducted me into a side room. He read from the notes.

'May I see the notes?' I asked.

'That is not allowed.'

'Well, can I see the X-rays?' He considered a moment and then handed me the envelope. I took out the films. 'Is there a fluorescent screen?'

'I'm afraid not.'

Obviously the whole place was terrorized by the Professor. I burst into laughter.

'Are you telling me, Herr Doktor, that in this marvellously equipped German clinic there is not an X-ray viewing screen?'

'They are for private use,' he said.

'All right,' I replied. 'Forget it.'

I took the films and held them up on the glass pane of one of the windows. With a few sheets of flimsy typewriting paper I traced the outline of the bones and the fracture which remained un-united. I handed the plates back to him.

'You will see that this is going to be a long affair,' the doctor said. The traction seemed to me to have kept the fractured ends of the bone apart.

'Thank you,' I said. 'And may I now see the patient?'

'Professor Domrich,' he began.

I smiled and put an arm round the younger man's shoulder.

'I am quite sure, Doctor,' I said, 'that the Herr Professor has every confidence in you to act on his behalf and quite as well as himself. I shall be very grateful if you would take me to Miss Steppat. I know her. I have examined her before, and she is a very charming person. I have come all the way from London. Do you know London?'

The soft soap just worked. The doctor smiled.

'Yes, I know it quite well. I also know Oxford where I studied for a time.'

'So did I,' I beamed. 'So let's go and get this all over shall we?'

He gave a little bow.

'Very well, Herr Doctor. *Komm mit mich.*'

Ilsa Steppat was indeed a charming person. She smiled and was quite effusive in her welcome. She was a very heavy woman and had chronic bronchitis. Her arm was strapped into a splint holding it out at right angles.

'Are you in pain?' I asked her.

'It is very uncomfortable,' she said miserably. I asked the nurse to take off the dressings and bandages. She had a very swollen arm and the skin round the traction pin wounds was red and puffy. I didn't need to look any more.

When the doctor and I got outside her room I said, 'Aren't you worried about infection?'

'She is on antibiotics.'

'Thrombosis?'

'She is on anticoagulants.'

'And her bronchitis? Keeping her in bed?'

'It is a risk.'

'Look, it's not for me to question anything. Mine is merely a fact finding mission, but off the record do you always treat this fracture like this?'

There was a momentary pause.

'Herr Professor Domrich treats the fracture like this,' he said.

'Well doctor, thank you very much for your kind co-operation. Tell Herr Professor I was sorry not to meet him. Goodbye.'

We shook hands and I got a car back to the Kempinski and put through a call to the Assessors. I reported my findings and added that under the present treatment, though orthodox, Ilsa Steppat would indeed not be able to shoot for many weeks.

'Then what the hell do you suggest we do?'

'The only way is to get someone of international orthopaedic standing to come over and see her and argue it out with Domrich.'

'Who have you in mind?'

'There's only one person. Lipmann-Kessel. And he speaks fluent German. He was also at Arnhem and is an old friend of the Krauts.'

'OK. Can you organize that?'

'I think so.'

'Right, carry on Ronnie.'

The upshot was that Lipmann-Kessel went out to Berlin a few days later where he was met by Cubby Broccoli, the producer of the Bond films. Lippy met with the same sort of obstruction that I had experienced. It appeared that Professor Domrich was not in favour of a consultation.

Broccoli got round this by taking Lippy in as a friend. Two stern looking females stood on each side of the bed, also introduced as friends of the actress. Her arm was still in the abduction frame. Lippy examined her. The fracture remained un-united. It was suggested that if she were to fly to London, alternative treatment might give her the best chance of meeting the date for the location shooting. Otherwise Broccoli implied they'd have to write her out of the picture.

The wretched actress was in a terrible dilemma. She wanted to stay in her film part but certainly in the presence of the two ladies patriotism prevailed.

With great emotion she said she had perfect confidence in Professor Domrich, that Berlin was her home, and Germany was her country, and she would not leave the hospital. She then burst into tears.

Lippy came home, but Broccoli stayed on and had a talk with Domrich. In the end Domrich allowed Ilsa out of the splint long enough for the shots, but insisted on accompanying his patient to the location and replacing the splint each evening. All his expenses and fees were paid. I believe these were a very considerable sum. Ilsa eventually recovered.

I suppose this time you could say it was game, set and match to the Germans.

15 'Flashback'

During the fifties and into the sixties as my practice grew, my nose was kept well down to the medical grindstone. But the muse still tugged incessantly at my sleeve. I was at an age where energy seems unbounded. I usually started out to see cases all over Greater London at eight-thirty in the morning driving ever more powerful cars, and returning at five to see some more patients. About eight I had dinner at home or we went out to eat two or sometimes three times a week. I was then capable of starting writing about ten-thirty and continuing to one-thirty or even two in the morning before going to bed. I was producing enough medical reports to keep two secretaries and one shorthand typist busy.

It was a mad routine and I was pushing myself to the limit. To ease the burden I engaged a driver. After one week, he gave notice. I asked why.

'Too much bleeding 'ard work.'

'But I usually do the driving and then all the medical work as well.'

'That's your lookout mate,' he said as he took his wages. It was an attitude in this country the years were to develop with the destructive social revolution that was taking place.

Another man objected to my calling him Jenkins, instead of Mister Jenkins.

'But I often call my friends by their surname,' I said.

'Well, to me it's *Mister* Jenkins.'

I gave him a week's wages out of my pocket, said goodbye and took over the steering wheel.

Finally, I had an American lady who said she had driven Eisenhower during the war. She went across a red light on Lavender Hill and a lorry nearly killed us.

After that I felt better being on my own.

At weekends I entertained the children. We visited all the well-known sights and museums in London, went to the cinema, and I actually climbed the Monument commemorating the Fire of London no less than four times. It is one of the stiffest exercise tolerance tests I know.

In June 1950 a comedy *Taking Things Quietly*, about an unholy alliance between a young barrister and Britain's oldest burglar (retired), was tried out by the Sunday Night Repertory Players at Wyndham's. On the Monday morning it had startlingly good reviews. The one I liked most was by Patrick Gibbs in *The Daily Telegraph*. He wrote 'This situation, beautifully developed and elaborated, yields up much laughter, the lines too, not to mention the characters, for Mr. Thorn has an eye for the ridiculous which conceals, as it should, a technically excellent piece of comic construction.'

The play was bought for transfer to the West End in the second interval by a management called Reanco, but I wish I had been able to wait until the Monday because there were five other offers, one being from the famed H. M. Tennent and Co. But as so often happens the iron was not struck when hot and the management dithered about changing the cast and the producer and waiting for the right theatre. After about six months of anguished waiting I was at last called to a casting meeting at the offices in the Strand.

The first question I was asked by E. P. Clift was,

'Mr. Thorn, who do you think should play the butler?'

'The burglar you mean?'

'No, the butler.'

'But there isn't a butler in my play,' I said.

He shuffled some papers on his desk and then to my astonishment asked,

'What's the name of your play?'

'*Taking Things Quietly*.'

He beamed at me benevolently.

'I'm most terribly sorry, old chap. I appear to have got the wrong author. I really must get round to reading your piece sometime.' He thrust out his hand. 'I'll be in touch.'

I left the room in a daze. They'd paid out money for an option, renewed it, and still hadn't read the damned thing. I passed the secretary in the outer office.

'My apologies, Mr. Thorn,' she said. 'I'm afraid it's my fault sending for you.'

'Does this often happen?' I asked. For answer she opened a cupboard which contained dozens of play scripts.

'Waiting for him to read,' she said.

Total disbelief was an understatement. I gave her a sickly smile and went down the stairs.

This omen was a forerunner of more disasters to come. Eventually Basil Radford was cast as the young barrister – at least thirty-odd years too old. I had to re-write his part cutting it down because he couldn't memorize long flowery speeches which were an essential part of the comedy.

When the play eventually came into the Ambassadors Theatre on 30 June 1951, after three weeks out of London, the stage manager and his lady assistant had had a tiff and were not speaking to one another. Ten minutes before the end of the last act, Eliot Makeham (who was superb as the burglar) couldn't open a door to get out of the set in the hurry which the action demanded because the button on the door had not been released in the second interval. Perfect professional that he was, he ad-libbed a line, 'Never mind, I'll go through the window.' This he did, tripped on a cable and brought down the flood-light illuminating the back drop with a flash and a resounding crash. The Humphrey Perkins Old Students Dramatic Society couldn't have done it better. The audience were throwing themselves about with laughter for entirely the wrong reason.

This catastrophe had the effect of drying Basil Radford up for at least two minutes. He kept opening his mouth but no sound came forth. The point of the scene was totally lost in promptings from other members of the cast. When Basil hesitantly said the final curtain line, sounds of argument about whose fault everything was were audible from backstage in the stalls.

Basil repeated the last line somewhat louder but still the curtain stayed up. There was more ad-libbing and eventually it slowly descended. I did the same inside the Author's box.

The next morning I was mortified to read how good all the cast were, but it was a pity the author had no idea how to end his play.

It ran for ten days, and was one of the last at the Ambassadors before *The Mousetrap* began its thirty-year marathon. I went to the first night and perhaps can be forgiven for expressing loudly in the foyer, during an interval, my considered opinion 'Well, this certainly won't run.'

I was not entirely desolate though because while waiting for *Taking Things Quietly* to come on, Amanda was born in the London Clinic on 18 September 1950 and on 25 September *They're Open!*, the book on beer drinking I had written with Roger Frisby, was at last published by the Harvill Press, I believe the twentieth publisher I had submitted it to. The book sold at Christmas for years and years. On 25 October 1950 the Repertory Players again tried their luck with me and did *Personal Call* on a Sunday at the Comedy, but it just failed to transfer.

The Ambassadors débâcle had taught me a lot about the theatre. A production, however prestigious, always hangs upon flimsy threads (totally out of control of the playwright), which can snap and mean disaster. But writing plays, if there is a modicum of talent, is a drug and a habit as strong as smoking or pot. I couldn't give it up, nor could I avoid the trials and tribulations the activity brings with it.

My next venture was a play called *The Love Machine* about a man's wife who falls in love with a TV announcer. She drives her husband to desperate measures to eliminate his rival on the box, by kidnapping him and impersonating him on the small screen. Alexander Doré directed it and it played a week at Leicester before a West End management bought it and took it out on a sixteen week pre-London tour. Diane Hart and Griffith Jones did their best, but the management went bust and it never came in. The best thing I got out of it was that at least I'd had one play performed at the Shakespeare Theatre, Stratford, albeit to miserably thin houses.

An old schoolfriend John Rhys, who did the special effects, got Peter Hoare to put on my new one *Bed of Roses* for a week at Frinton Summer Theatre, Jack Watling playing the main part. Nothing happened to it subsequently except that Evans Plays published it.

But I was getting the message so I turned to doing some film scripts and books. At least with the latter, I felt what was down in black and white couldn't be mucked about by anybody – except of course bad presentation and promotion by the publisher.

On 18 March 1952 Thelma bore me another daughter, Vanessa, and for a few years family delights took over.

In June 1957 a book about the antics of *au pairs* – as parents we had worked through nearly four a year on average – called *Upstairs and Downstairs* was published by Neville Spearman. It was an undoubted success, going into Pan paperback here, and being published in America. Betty Box filmed the book and I believe made quite a lot of money out of it. It launched Claudia Cardinale and Mylene Demongeot and the music and songs went into the charts.

About this time in the middle of a very harassed and busy afternoon, I had a call from the Cornhill Insurance Company, and the Claims Manager, a delightfully canny Scotsman named Bruce, asked to speak to me. He was also a dry wit of no mean talent which, as well as the call being taken while a patient stood behind the screen with his clothes off, may have contributed to my flippant response.

'Can you please tell me, Dr. Thorn,' he asked, 'what would be the fee for your examining a patient in New York for us?'

'Oh, er, the usual ten guineas,' I said.

'Ten guineas?' he exclaimed. 'You're not serious?'

A sound of impatience came from behind the screen.

'Oh, well,' I said to Bruce. 'As we're old friends I could make it seven.'

'I'll ring you back,' he said.

I examined the patient, dictated the report to Mary Cohen and the phone went again.

'Hello doctor. Bruce here. We'd like you to do the job for us. When can you go?'

I then realized how serious he was.

'Ah yes,' I faltered. 'Well of course that fee . . .'

'Ach,' he said, 'a bargain's a bargain, doctor, you know that.'

'Yes,' I replied.

'All expenses paid in addition naturally.'

My mind began to work furiously.

'Right,' I said. 'Seven guineas for the examination and report, but I hate flying so I want First Class return on the *Queen Elizabeth* and I should need to stay at the Waldorf Astoria.'

'That's more like it,' Bruce laughed. 'I wouldn't be asking you to go for us if I thought you were daft enough to charge a silly fee without strings. Done. I'll send you the papers laddie.' He rang off.

I left ten days later on the old *Queen Elizabeth*. As I looked up at the towering sides of the vessel, I was as excited as a schoolboy. I recalled the last time I had been in Southampton was when at the age of five while on holiday from Ryde, IOW, I had coughed my way round the *Aquetania* on a sightseeing trip with my parents, who had no idea that I must have spread infection throughout the ship, until the next day when I went to bed with whooping cough.

The colossal size of a ship like the *Queen Elizabeth* is overawing. Though I only had an inside cabin it was airconditioned and eminently comfortable, and of course it had the first class service by stewards who seemed to belong to the world of the twenties. The music played by the orchestra in the grand lounge – Coward, Berlin, Porter, Novello – strengthened the atmosphere. The morning cosseting on the boat deck with rugs and cushions and bowls of steaming bouillon was from another age. A passenger in blazer and white flannels looking quite like Jack Buchanan actually asked another voyager who had not found a seat, 'Would you like a deck chair, old boy?'

I found it impossible to go to bed early the first night and stayed up until we moored at Cherbourg to pick up the French passengers. I saw some very chic ladies wrapped in furs against the cold come up the gangway, their cabin trunks having been stowed aft, and I thought nostalgically of the Comtesse, and Elie, and Rolande and wondered where they were.

The great *Queen* eventually turned her bows westward towards the swell and the rain and the wind of the Atlantic. I had a last brandy, settled into my bunk between the crisp linen sheets and blessed the Cornhill Insurance Company.

I awoke with a start in the night. There seemed an uncanny quietness about everything except the unmistakable sound of water sloshing around on the floor of the cabin. In a panic I switched on the light. My suitcase and medical bag were awash. My God, I thought, we're sinking. Why haven't I been told? No running footsteps, no booming siren from the funnels. The boats had been lowered and I'd never heard the call to abandon ship. I'd just been forgotten! In a half sleeping state I put a foot on to the floor. It was real water all right. I pushed every bell push I could find and bellowed 'Steward!' at the top of my voice.

Within five seconds one appeared.

'What's happened? Are we sinking?' I asked idiotically.

'Dear oh dear oh dear. No, we are not sir,' came the reassuring reply.

'Then where's all the water coming from?'

'A leak in your lavatory, sir. I do apologize. On behalf of the Captain, of course. Now you get back into bed, sir, and we'll have this cleared up in no time. The plumber will be straight along. And don't worry about your luggage, we'll have that dried out in no time too. I am very sorry about this, sir.'

In ten minutes the job was done. I was given a free glass of whisky and the next day a further apology from the Purser. All really rather trivial but I slept well from then on, and am rather stupidly proud of the water mark which can still be seen round my old medical bag.

On the trip over to the States I met Eric Weiss, the chairman of Foseco-Minsep, with whom I had dinner each evening in the celebrated Verandah Grill. After four days I was sick of the look of caviar supplied in unlimited quantities. At lunch the first day a sprightly mischievous-eyed man in his late forties at one of the round tables looked at my Oxford University tie and stated casually,

'Ah, I see the book and triple crown. Fletcher-Cooke, Dr. Thorn?'

'Yes,' I said, 'but how do you . . .?'

'It's all on the printed passenger list, I was at Teddy Hall. And you were at?'

'Merton,' I replied and we dived into the salmon mousse together. I discovered that John, after being as he put it, one of the Emperor's guests in a Japanese POW Camp for three years, had been Governor of Cyprus and later acting Governor of Tanganyika and was then on his way to the United Nations in charge of the Trusteeship Council. Over the years we became intimate friends.

I also encountered Winsor French, an American columnist. As I had taken the precaution to put six copies of the just published *Upstairs and Downstairs* in my case, I gave him one and later he kindly wrote a glowing review of me and the book in the Cleveland Press, when I was published in the States. I also presented two copies to the Ship's library. Word went round and that was the nearest I ever got to being an ephemeral minor celebrity. It was a heady feeling and my confidence began busting out all over. This was slightly dimmed when I started chatting to an attractive blonde at the bar. She told me she was unmarried and from Texas, so I said, 'I suppose you own an oil-well too?'

With a deadpan expression she replied,

'No, honey. I own ten.'

The conversation never got back on its feet.

The impact of the Big Apple has been written about a good deal, and I suppose it always will be. The only way to approach New York for the first time is undoubtedly from the sea. The magic rise on the horizon of that faery towering city is more expressive of man's ingenuity and creative virile aspirations than any place on earth. It *is* the New World; it is the shape of the twentieth century. What new evils it contains are no greater than the old ones it has left behind. It is Man. Us. Now.

Maurice Hodgson, an old friend from Merton doing a stint for ICI in New York (before much later becoming chairman), met me at the dockside. Having settled me in to the Waldorf we went out for some food and then to Times Square. I stood and gawped like any simple country boy. Unlike the London I knew so well the lights seemed to go up as far as they spread horizontally. A huge effigy of Marilyn announcing her film *Niagara* sat atop a real waterfall twenty storeys high which sprayed the sidewalks and across Broadway. Next to it a huge mouth puffed a twenty-foot wide smoke ring advertising Lucky Strike. Hodge and I looked at each other and laughed. What sort of people were they? How could they do such things? We laughed our way into several bars, dark comfortable and hidden away, all with padded edges in front of the stools, designed presumably to prevent injuries to the ribs as the customers slumped alcoholically forward. In each bar was a resident drunk, unconscious but unmolested, it appeared, for several days. Though speaking English in this strange world, I felt more of a foreigner than if I were in Rome, speaking no Italian.

I began to move differently, using my shoulders as organs of locomotion. My request to the cab driver,

'Would you mind taking me to –' was cut short by:

'Where to buddy?' I soon learnt all that was necessary was to get in the vehicle and snarl, '527 East 25th'. We whooshed away before I had finished the sentence. My thanks to the lift operator on reaching my floor in the hotel was met with a startled smile and the surprised remark, 'You're welcome, sir.'

On instructions, the morning after I arrived, about 8.00 a.m. I called the doctor's office who was the first consultant with whom I had to see the patient I had come to examine. Instead of the usual response I would have got in London, 'I'm sorry, who did you say you were . . .? No he's not in . . . No I don't know when he'll be back,' I was greeted welcomingly by the silvery-voiced receptionist. 'Good morning Dr. Thorn. We were expecting your call. You arrived last night on the *Queen Elizabeth*. I hope you had a good trip. The doctor will meet you at the hospital at 9.00 a.m. Have a good day.'

As I sped up Park Avenue in a yellow cab to the hospital I wondered how the consultation was going to turn out. The only other occasion I had been abroad on a medico-legal claim for an insurance company was to Turin some years before.

I had been sent the fifteen-page translation of a report on a lady who had broken her leg (this time a 'Tib and Fib') by a Professore Dottore. We met at the patient's house. The Professore was a man of sartorial splendour in his mid-fifties. He was wearing a white silk suit, a magenta tie and perfume. While I examined the patient in her bedroom he perched himself on an elegant commode. His short legs swung back and forth some inches from the floor exposing magenta socks and black and white handmade shoes which would have undoubtedly rung the bell at Lloyds. He spent the time as I worked polishing his nails with great concentration.

I had taken the precaution of hiring my own interpreter from Thomas Cook's. As I made my observations and measurements I compared them with the figures the Professore had recorded in his report. The discrepancies were so considerable that it might have been a different patient.

'Please tell the Professore I find the leg is shortened by only 1.5 centimetres. He says it is 9.0 centimetres.'

The interpreter conveyed the message. The Professore gave a shrug and smiled at me agreeably.

'Does he agree with my figure?'

The Professore nodded happily.

'*Si, si, Signor*,' he said to me.

This procedure was repeated with all my other findings.

The examination completed, the Professore shook one of mine with both his hands, and the patient in virtually biblical fashion threw away her sticks, leapt off the bed and led us into a dining room where her family of ten was introduced. With much hilarity and vino we all sat down to a large meal. The interpreter and I left the building about three hours later. I paid him his fee. Everyone seemed happy, especially the insurance company as I had reduced the claim by a very large amount.

In New York the patient was an elderly multi-millionaire

newspaper proprietor who had hired several rooms in the hospital for me to carry out the examination. He had fractured both femurs on a visit to England while a passenger in a hire-car, insured by the Cornhill. He had been treated suitably and shipped back to the States in plasters. All that was required to be done was remove the plaster and give him physiotherapy and rehabilitation. His total bill in London was under £1,000. In the three months after his return to New York the medical fees had risen to £20,000. What would have taken two hours in London for consultation, took me five days in New York with seven doctors. Everyone, for safety's sake, had come into the act, as well as the orthopaedic surgeon – radiologists, physicians, cardiologists, pathologists, genito-urinary men and a geriatrician. I thought one guinea for each consultation?

The orthopod met me at the top of the steps of the hospital with effusive greetings. Proudly he showed me a large indicator system with lights that ran vertically and horizontally to locate any doctor in the building.

'I don't know if you have this system,' he said. 'I have just arrived and all I have to do is to push this button by my name here.'

He pushed the button. Nothing happened. He pushed it again, with the same result.

'What the hell's going on around here?' he exclaimed. 'My circuit will have to be checked out.'

I couldn't resist the comment.

'We would have a wooden slip with your name painted on it. When you came in at the end of the slip would be the word "Out". You would shove it along and the word at the other end would appear "In". It doesn't often go wrong.'

He perceptibly scowled at me and we went to see the patient. After an hour or so the patient had us served with sandwiches and coffee.

It was then my turn to see the radiologist and I was conducted to the basement. A pile of X-rays several inches thick were presented for my inspection.

'I don't know if you're used to viewing Skiagrams on a daylight viewing screen. You're probably still on the fluorescent ones, but we find the daylight method, especially with skeletal shots, shows up the fine bone trabeculae much better.'

He took me to a row of glass panels. These turned out to be windows giving on to concave matt-white backgrounds. The light came down from the street above.

I worked laboriously through all the films of which I thought eighty per cent were unnecessary or irrelevant. Then I asked my American colleague if he had a 100 watt bulb.

'Bulb?'

'Light bulb.'

'Oh, a globe.'

'Yes, I find it simple but useful as an intensifier for looking at trabeculae.'

'Sure, sure,' he said, 'if that's what you want.'

A bulb was produced. He looked at the film over my shoulder.

'The left fracture is completely united but the right is still only in the thick callus stage. Do you agree?' I asked.

He moved the bulb back and forth.

'I certainly do,' he said, then laughed and shook his head in amusement. 'Well, what do you know? Just a hundred watt globe.'

I had a sneaking suspicion that the next day his department was going to be lavishly furnished with simple light bulbs.

My next surprise was an invitation by the patient to go to his flat so that he could show me how he was combating his disability. He had dispensed with sticks and used an overhead railway with handles which whizzed him from room to room rather like the old fashioned cashier systems in drapers' shops. He also demonstrated two huge wooden contraptions like scissors so that he could stand in his trousers and shoot them up his legs without having to bend his hips. He took me down to his Cadillac the side of which had been cut away. A ramp came down. His wheel chair mounted it, rotated, automatically clamped into place beside his chauffeur and we were off to lunch.

I had the utmost admiration for that man. He demonstrated all the great American traits of invention, perseverance, refusal of defeat and 'get up and go'. Sadly, of course, by this adaptability he was reducing the value of his claim. I think I saved the Cornhill many thousands. But it was such a refreshing change from the British malingerers.

While in New York perhaps my most memorable delight was being able for the price of a beer to go down to the Metropole on Broadway and hear some of my jazz folk heroes in the flesh. I remember particularly Tony Pastor's biting tenor sax, Cozy Cole's firework displays on the drums and Mr. Jesus Christ Higginbotham on a mellow slide-horn.

Someone I had met on the boat coming over had asked me to meet him for a drink one night at the Barclay Bar. I assumed that it was the Berkeley, duly arrived there, and waited for him to appear. As I waited, a Bostonian sitting next to me put down three large Martinis in about ten minutes. Then he suddenly rolled up his eyes and fell off his stool backwards. I heard his skull crack on the floor. I leapt up to help him but a strong barman's hand restrained me.

'Leave him alone, he's dead.'

'But I'm a doctor . . .'

'So what can you do? Leave him alone.'

I watched horrified. There was a corpse at my feet and I was doing nothing. The sounds of the bar continued normally. Then suddenly the man got up, brushed himself down and said,

'Excuse me,' and left the bar.

'What did I tell you, doc?' grinned the barman.

In less than five minutes the Bostonian returned, sat on his stool, smiled at me amiably and gave his order.

'Martini.'

'Coming up, Sir,' the barman winked at me. Whatever the Hollywood films had taught me, they seemed suddenly an understatement of the real thing.

A couple of fags and a girl came in and were immediately extremely friendly to me. I was not surprised as in the States it is impossible not to get into a conversation in a very short time.

I found at first it took a native about one minute before he asked 'You a Britisher?' After two and a half weeks I had lengthened the period to seven minutes. I also discovered that early on in any encounter the direct question 'What do you make?' would come up. At first I was confused and replied that I didn't make anything, I was a doctor. The answer sought for was how many dollars a year did I earn. I used to give various answers and found that the response friendly or otherwise was directly linked to the amount stated. The fags and girl bought me a drink, of which I had never heard before.

'Now isn't that the most wonderful drink you've ever tasted?' I was asked.

I certainly didn't think so but in order to be polite I gave my opinion.

'Yes . . . it's not altogether unpleasant.'

'What sort of answer is that? Do you like it or don't you like it?'

I was learning the hazards of the double negative.

'I like it,' I said firmly.

'Give him another one, Joe.'

My protests were brushed aside. Things seemed to be getting friendly. My next invitation was to join the three round at somebody's place for a party. The second unnameable was mellowing me considerably. Obviously the person I was supposed to be meeting would not show up now.

'Well,' I said when a pink slip of folded paper was pushed along the bar to me by a man a few stools away. He must have been six foot five. I opened the note. It read,

'Go easy friend. J. D. Bodge Room 804.'

I looked across at him. Without smiling he shook his head slowly from side to side.

I was still sober enough to recognize a warning and extricated myself from my three new friends, who shrugged and left the room. Puzzled, I went up and sat next to Bodge.

'You're a Britisher,' he said. 'Don't know this bar?'

'No.'

'Well, I hate to see someone taken for a ride. If you'd have gone with them, they'd have had the shirt off your back. Drink?'

'No, thanks,' I said.

'Do you play poker?'

'I have done,' I replied.

'Great. Well, if you come up in the elevator to the eighth floor in ten minutes, there's a nice friendly little school starting.'

He flipped the brim of his stetson and lumbered out of the bar.

It dawned on me I was in a big pool full of what are known as the real alligators. I paid my check, shot out into the street and got back to the Waldorf as quickly as I could. Going home on the *Queen Mary* I stuck to Bingo. I also had a crew-cut on board, which did not suit me, but made certain ladies want to rub my head just for the feel of the bristles. Thelma walked right past me on the platform when she met the boat train at Waterloo. Obviously I was never going to be the same again.

16 Daily Rushes

As the children grew older, family holidays became more and more the major events of the year, not to mention the major expense. Mummy took most of the strain of these annual ordeals. Occasionally we took the *au pair* or 'mother's hindrance' to complicate the expedition and get extra laughs.

I was in charge of bookings and transport. Thelma had an uncanny knack of finding a perfectly logical reason for changing our destination, and usually at the last minute, the manner of our travel. I was kept on the jump booking and re-booking bookings. If anything ultimately went wrong, I carried the can of complaints which had to be dealt with. So before we had the additional complication of children I had learnt the sort of thing to expect.

The first time I took Thelma to Paris she was ecstatic about the hotel, which was quite a grand one. After our bags had been put in our room, which was large and splendidly furnished, and the door had closed on the porters, Thelma inspected the fully tiled bathroom, tested the water supply and the bidet, and checked the springing of the bed. Her lovely face took on a slightly disappointed air.

'Pretty good, eh?' I remarked hopefully, and began to unpack.

'I can't stay in this room,' she said quietly.

'Why on earth not?'

'Brown. I don't like brown. The curtains are brown and the bed is brown.'

'Well, the carpet's not,' I said.

'Brown depresses me, darling. You remember that brown suit you had?'

'Yes?'

'Well, I hated it.'

'I never knew that, what happened to it?'

'I threw it away. And I can't stay in this room, so you needn't unpack. We shall have to move to another one.'

'Look, sweetie,' I said, 'this is a perfectly good room. And I'm not going to make a fool of myself by asking for another one.'

'Then I am,' said Thelma and picked up the phone. 'Would you send the manager up please?' she asked in dulcet tones.

'Now Thelma, I'm having nothing to do with this.'

'Then hide, darling. Skulk in the bathroom.'

And that is what I did, keeping the door ajar so that I could overhear the conversation. When the manager arrived, Thelma charmed the pants off him. It took her about three minutes to get him to assent to everything she said.

'But of course, Madame, I agree with you absolutely. *Brun* is a very depressing colour. You are completely right. You cannot possibly stay in this awful room. We shall change you immediately. You would like something light and gay?'

'Oh yes, that's just what I'd like,' purred Thelma.

'I have exactly the room. I will send the porters up for the baggage.'

He disappeared soundlessly. I came out of the bathroom, my mouth sagging open.

'You see?' smiled Thelma. 'No difficulty at all.'

We were moved to the top floor to a pink and white room with a view over the Arc de Triomphe. I tipped the porters for the second time.

'This is just wonderful,' exclaimed Thelma. 'You *must* agree this is quite a different thing altogether. One feels quite uplifted up here.'

I nodded dumbly. It was the best suite in the hotel with a salon and a balcony. I looked at the little card on the back of the door which told me the price. It was exactly three times as expensive as the other one.

'Aren't you glad, darling?' she asked and put her arms round my neck and kissed me.

'I can't stand fucking pink,' was all I could think of to say.

At London Airport in the departure lounge Amanda succeeded in showering some Coca Cola over her mother's new silk two-piece. Thelma did not conceal her fury: she announced she couldn't possibly travel with stains all over her clothes. Our luggage was on the plane. We would have to go home, change and we would go on the next one – next day. Thelma was a very chic-looking lady.

Amanda was in tears. Vanessa did her saucer-eyed act of perfect innocence. Fortunately, the stains began to dry out.

'Quite a nice effect,' I said feebly.

But it was nip and tuck that we eventually boarded the plane for Algeçiras.

On another holiday at the Cap Estel at Eze-bord-de-Mer after one meal and a bite on the finger she received from a little Danish boy called Knut, Vanessa refused to eat any more food.

'In that case,' I said, 'there's no point in your sitting at the table.'

She got down with dignity, and whether in protest at Amanda's insistence on trying everything on the gourmet menu, Vanessa used to parade up and down the terrace in her bikini scowling at all the dining guests.

After three days of this performance, Thelma remarked Vanessa was looking decidedly thinner.

'You're a doctor, why don't you do something?' she pestered me. 'She'll be ill if she doesn't eat.'

'Might even die of starvation,' said Amanda finishing a huge plate of profiteroles.

'Well, *you* certainly won't,' I said irritably.

'It's ruining the holiday,' went on Thelma, 'And beginning to make *me* feel ill,' as she disposed of the last spoonful of *fraises des bois* and cream.

'Allow me to know how to treat anorexia, will you?' I said. 'If we ignore the whole thing and make no comment, eventually Vanessa will sit down and gobble up everything.'

But Vanessa didn't. At the end of the fourth day a plump middle-aged motherly English woman approached me. She pointed to Vanessa and asked,

'Excuse me,' she said, 'but that *is* your daughter isn't it?'

'My younger one,' I said.

'Well, I know it's none of my business but I've had five children and if that child of yours doesn't eat soon, she's going to be ill. I think you should take her to a doctor.'

'I *am* a doctor,' I glared.

'Oh? Oh, I'm extremely sorry. I didn't know. Excuse me.'

She went off and we had no further conversation. But as we approached the end of our first week I did have a conversation with Vanessa and attempted to get her to eat some bread and butter and some fruit. Fortunately she was drinking a lot of milk and occasionally swallowed a chocolate, but to everything else she shook her head.

I called a family conference.

'I have decided to cut the holiday short – we're not enjoying it and I refuse to pay full pension terms if we're not eating the food. I've cancelled the rooms for the second week, and we're leaving tomorrow morning. So everybody had better start packing. I'm going to get the car filled up with petrol.'

There were howls of rage from Amanda who suggested her sister should be sent home by plane on her own. Vanessa looked out to sea with a dreamy expression. Thelma, for once, had no words to offer but sighed resignedly.

As we were having a last drink in the bar prior to our departure, in a small still voice, Vanessa said, 'Could I have some bread and cheese? And I wouldn't mind a strawberry ice.'

These were brought and Vanessa wolfed them down greedily while Amanda and her mother piled abuse on her. Vanessa paid no attention whatsoever. I slipped away to the Reception to see if I could get our rooms back, but it was high season and they were already re-let. Taking the Guide Michelin I phoned six other hotels and pensions but there was not a room to be had.

I went back to the bar.

'I'm sorry,' I said, 'but everywhere's full up. We've just got to drive home.'

'But why should Mummy and I suffer just because of *her*?' said Amanda.

'Hard cheese,' I said.

We loaded the car and drove along the coast towards Nice before turning up the road back to Grasse. As we went through Juan-les-Pins, I stopped outside the Grand Hotel.

'I'll try one more time. There might just have been a cancellation, but I doubt it. So everyone stay in the car.'

I went up to the girl at the reception desk. Her face was vaguely familiar.

'Hello, Doctor Thorn,' she said. 'Do you remember me, Yvette? I was your *au pair* three years ago.'

'Why yes, I remember.'

'And 'ow is Mrs. Thorn and Amanda and Vanessa?'

'They're in the car outside.'

'I would love to see them. Have you had a good holiday?'

I gave a hollow laugh and told her what had happened, and added, 'I know it's a silly request but I suppose you haven't got two double rooms?'

Yvette shook her pretty head sadly. 'We are completely booked monsieur, I am afraid.'

'I thought you might be,' I replied.

I turned to go away but she briefly put a hand on mine while she gave the same information to two other couples at the desk. When they had gone she winked at me.

'*Attendez, Monsieur le docteur.*'

Yvette spoke rapidly down the desk phone and then turned to me again with a charming smile. 'We always keep some accommodation for personal friends of the management. My 'usband owns the hotel.'

So we had our second week after all. But the holiday was not over. When we reached Boulogne and I went to drive the car off the car-carrier train, the engine wouldn't start. Eventually my Jag was ignominiously pushed off and left stranded on the quayside. My wife and daughters stood by as silent spectators while I tried everything I knew under the bonnet to no avail. The car ferry sailed away. The look of sad contempt in three pairs of female eyes is an unnerving experience. Eventually a French mechanic in traditional beret arrived. He muttered incoherently and in one minute flat had the engine running. We caught the next boat and arrived home at Wimpole Street late and hungry. The final blow fell on me like a sledge hammer. I couldn't find the flat key and Thelma hadn't got hers. After another two hours a locksmith came, bored a hole in the door and got us in. When he had gone, I asked Thelma. 'I suppose there isn't any food?'

'Of course there isn't,' she said. 'But I expect there is at the Dorchester.'

It was a very expensive holiday.

During all this orgy of domestic masochism I managed to write my first full-length novel *The Full Treatment*. Paul Scott of David Higham Associates sold it to Heinemann but owing to a printing strike in 1959 it was not published until March 1960. Pan brought it out in paperback in July 1963.

In the meantime Richard Gregson had sold the film rights to Columbia with Val Guest directing. Diane Cilento, Ronald Lewis, Françoise Rosay and Claude Dauphin were the stars.

I was engaged to write the screenplay with Val Guest, making it my first film collaboration. Val's vast experience in the job of writing and directing soon made me realize that any difference of opinion of mine on the dialogue or script was subject to his absolute veto, because he was directing as well as writing. I also realized, as I had earlier on some of the Betty Box and Ralph Thomas productions in the 'Doctor' series, that most of what you write is altered or scrapped or finally left lying on the cutting room floor. It is not really a game for authors except for the money. *The Full Treatment* proved a valuable experience in this respect. On the whole Val and I got on extremely well, and we have remained friends up to the present time.

I had set the action in London and my obsessively favourite holiday area, the Riviera, and we had an intense two weeks on location in and near Cannes. I spent a lot of time watching the shooting and learnt still more about film making. Naturally, I had passed all the cast fit at the pre-production medicals. The atmosphere on location was tense, involved and the overcurrents of a power struggle all too obvious. Bryan Forbes's recent novel *The Re-write Man* describes and develops this situation that he knows so well with consummate skill and inside knowledge.

For the period of the location I took the family with me and ensconced them nearby at the 'Pins et Plage' at Agay. So that Thelma and I could have time off to ourselves and leave the children safely on the beach, and guarded at night I took Grazia with us, this time an Italian *au pair* of voluptuous proportions. No sooner had she arrived than she announced she could not go on the beach during her period. This knocked the first few days on the head. She then demanded that she should take a week off to go to Rome to see her mother on the excuse of some complicated family reason. I refused to let her go as she was being paid to be with Amanda and Vanessa and that's why she was with us.

'But I must see my mother,' she said.

'Then tell her to come here,' I foolishly replied.

In two days I had an elderly lady dressed in black staying in the little hotel with us for the rest of the holiday – all, of course, at my expense. It was a pretty disastrous arrangement and I saw the proceeds of the sale of my film rights being washed away inexorably like the sand of the *Mer Mediterranée*.

Nevertheless, Val got all the shots in the can without a day overshooting and the film had its première in London in February 1961 to mixed reviews. Surprisingly, after retitling it to *Stop Me Before I Kill*, the picture did much better in the States. I was most pleased with the review in *The New York Times* by Howard Thompson who said 'The British have concocted a snug tautly-strung thriller . . . there are no complaints for the dialogue has a nice cutting edge, the tempo and photography are crisp . . . Mr.

Guest's package is a small one, but trim and adroitly told. The contents are well worth waiting for.'

On the strength of this, my next novel *Second Opinion* was published by Heinemann in 1961 and Macmillan in New York in 1962. It went into British and U.S. paperback and was translated all over the place. The *Los Angeles Times* said of the book 'The characters are expertly drawn, complex enough to allow contention and conflict'. Someone else wrote '. . . nearly as good as Graham Greene'. But of course not quite.

Peter Rogers bought the film rights and I wrote the screenplay. But we were hitting the slump in the film industry, with TV taking its toll of cinema box offices. The script still lies on a shelf somewhere in Pinewood gathering dust.

The Twin Serpents was also published by Macmillan in New York in 1965 after Heinemann published it over here in 1964. *The Twin Serpents* was the Dollar Book Club choice for December 1965 and ran into 400,000 copies. It had a wonderful success. I've sold the film option four times, but the picture is yet to be made.

The point comes when an author stops writing for a time and takes a breather and a look at himself and what he wants to write in the future.

I think this was triggered off for me by my father's death in June 1965. He and my mother had come to live in a small top flat in Upper Wimpole Street after his retirement from Humphrey Perkins at Barrow. He busied himself with marking 'A' level papers and other papers regularly for a Correspondence College to eke out his pension. He was a happy man and encouraged me all my life in everything I tried to do. Idleness was a crime to him and his example undoubtedly spurred me on. He was marvellously well attended by Walter Somerville, the cardiologist. He definitely prolonged my father's life, and became a close friend and mentor of mine.

One evening my father was marking some maths papers sitting in the armchair in his flat. Suddenly he put the papers and his blue marking pencil down, and said, 'I think I'll just have a rest for a minute.'

He closed his eyes and in a few seconds he was dead.

The shock of his going and the anguish of his absence from my life affected me for a number of years. It still does. My mother lived on. Her death didn't occur for another thirteen years. But from the day of my father's funeral, she began to shrink and wither before my eyes in spite of all my efforts to console and support her. The final sight of her dead wizened little body wrung my heart unbearably but I remember her always as she was, perhaps most when she was so lovely and gay and used to come and see me at Shrewsbury.

These close personal events took the steam out of my literary efforts and I sought consolation in the growing up of my own children. They both went to Queen's College in Harley Street. Amanda went to Cambridge and got a good degree in Classics and then Law. She qualified as a solicitor but after a time gave it up to get married. Vanessa was a secretary first of the Dean of a Law School in Grays Inn Road and later of the Regius Professor of Medicine at Oxford. She married before Amanda. They both have children of their own.

After Thelma and I had been married for twenty-five years she left me and married Raymond Balfour. It was a divorce without acrimony and I have visited them several times since. They live in Fairford in Gloucestershire.

I bought a fifteenth-century cottage in Burford before this happened, and which I loved for a number of years. (The bathroom was an exotic affair, known in the town as Ronnie's folly.) But I lost the cottage in the end to Halina when we were divorced early in 1982.

While at Burford I did a lot of painting at the weekends and started writing again. I miss the Cotswold countryside, especially the russet splendours of autumn there, and Alec and Joan Swann, good friends who lived next door at the old vicarage. But as yet I haven't had the guts to go back and look at Richards Cottage in the High Street and realize that some unknown person is living there, touching the beams, stoking the fire and basking in the summer in the walled garden from which you can just see the spire of the church. But I will go back, I know. One day before I die.

In 1967 I gave up smoking – for the first time and kept it up for seven years. I know that the loss of the consolation was also a factor in making me quite unable to write for a long time. I had made many previous short-lived attempts without success. Giving up changes the personality. Whatever the methods, the tricks, the hypnotism, the substitutes, I'm convinced in the end the only sure reason for stopping is when fear is greater than desire.

When patients ask me how they can stop the habit, I find that I can give quite inadequate advice. The experience of giving up a lifelong way of life is traumatic and shattering. I can best express my feelings in a piece of verse I wrote about it which may help some people. I called it 'Ex-Smoker's Blues'.

'No thanks, I've given up'
A score of habit-years
When every pleasure was that much more
For a cigarette after, during or before.

148

To search the sad smokeless desert
For some other substitute knowing
There are no plants growing.

Grief recalling the first brief
Inhalation, the initial thoracic shock,
Stained fingers clutching at the heart
From then on, the comforting screen
Against the small hurt the larger pain
Subtle aid to clear thinking
Fiery wisdom stinking in the breath
Intellectuals' nervous prop
Creative excuse for 'Just can't stop'.

No longer the easing of little embarrassments
Celebration of great reliefs slight accomplishments
Small-hours panic-forage to find more
Pocket-pat to locate the solace if a bore
Should hold the evening's sway.
Avoiding now the eyes of friends still puffing
Reproaches. Act of denial treacherous
Bluffing the refusal through shock to trusted cronies
The mocking of the thrice-crowed cock.

New companions now from the other camp
Those who, prudish, boast they never have
Or worse the boast of him
Who did, and gave it up upon a whim
Without a pang or effort.
Fire and smoke
The first human stride from primeval dark
Degraded now to the request for a light
As bargaining starts
The spurious casualness of the tart's
Traditional approach
Fatal casualty's placebo for doom
The questioner's subversive weapon
In the interrogation room.
Learning the secret that original sin
Is a built-in
Carcinogen.

Yet if a sudden black catastrophe should strike,
Wife killed, children lost, reputation blown
Or when they tell me there's not long to go
I'll put on a brave transparent show
Of nonchalant unconcern
And send out for a pack, and drag deep down

The sweet lethal air once more
For if in Hell I shall burn
It will not deter me to ponder then
That there are no ashtrays in Heaven.

17 Recast

Like priests and undertakers a doctor is never off duty. The hours
are long, and pressure and fatigue often lead to embarrassments.

Long ago, when I was still in Weymouth Street, a patient was
sent in by my secretary in the midst of a heavy afternoon of cases. I
was running late, and this patient appeared to be French. He was
effusive and voluble. To reach the nub of the matter quickly I told
him to take off his shirt. He looked astonished and as he began
undoing his buttons he exclaimed 'But I am your *translateur!*'

'What do you mean?' I asked.

'The *translateur* of your *pièce L'Air des Montagnes.*'

My stethoscope end stopped on its way to his pectoral region as
the penny dropped. He had translated *Mountain Air* into French.
Hardly an action which called for a medical examination.

Early one morning after a hurried breakfast I had a consultation
with a Surgical Registrar in a hospital outpatient department. I sat
at a desk, the patient on one side, the registrar on the other.
Behind me were the Sister and a nurse. I was starting a cold. I
sneezed and took out my handkerchief from my breast pocket. A
piece of bacon came with it and fell on to the notes in front of me.
There was a short pause while we all looked at it. I felt an
explanation and apologies were going to hold things up and I was
in a hurry. So I took what I thought to be the quickest way out of
the embarrassment. I picked up the bacon and put it in my mouth
and crunched it somewhat noisily. Then I began taking the history
without further ado.

Working at speed has led me to give curious commands. I have
told a patient to take off his foot, meaning shoe and to one lady,
take off your head please, meaning hat.

Socially it is advisable as a doctor to keep a low profile. With
experience I have learnt like Tom in *The Glass Menagerie* to have
tricks in my mental pockets. At parties, it is necessary to fend off

requests for free medical advice, which can ruin many an evening's enjoyment. When details of symptoms are poured out gratuitously from guests I am occasionally driven to such dire and cruel remedies as saying,

'I don't like the sound of it. I should see your doctor first thing in the morning. Unless –'

'Unless what?'

'You can get to him tonight.'

This usually does the trick. Another jibe, once people know you are a doctor is, 'Why can't you doctors find a cure for the common cold?'

'There is one,' I often reply. 'Absolutely one hundred per cent guaranteed.'

'Oh? Please tell me.'

'Decapitation.'

This invariably provides a quick release.

One never treats relatives. Something always goes wrong. They never follow your advice. And you don't get a fee. Other doctors' wives are also a hazard. If you inject them you use the one in a thousand defective intramuscular needle which breaks off leaving a foreign body deep in a buttock. The upshot is a cheloidal operation scar after its removal, which is worn as a permanent reproach for life. Jean Paul Sartre said 'Hell is other people.' For doctors it is 'Hell is other doctors' wives.'

My long time colleague John Cronin, Labour M.P. for Loughborough for many years, a wit and an efficient surgeon had a general warning about relatives as patients. 'Receptacles for emotional blackmail, old boy.'

As I became more experienced, my opposing expert medical witnesses in court seemed to become less formidable. Some were masters of the craft. Charles Gray, consultant orthopod at the Royal Free, and a close friend, was impressive in the box. His devastating technique was the use of the one word answer. I recall his being asked what he thought of the opposing medical witness's opinion. He pondered carefully for a while and then replied, 'Nonsense.'

Others were not so successful. Judges hate verbose erudite answers. They also dislike any histrionic display. I remember one surgeon who in his enthusiasm to demonstrate the anatomy of a torn knee cartilage put his leg over the side of the box, and pulled up his trousers to show the surface anatomy of the cartilage. The judge thanked him and asked the Counsel if the witness was needed further, and ordered his release. This was not so easy. It took protracted efforts of the Usher and the Clerk to get the surgeon's leg back into the box. He was helped out of the court with a marked limp.

Archibald Jeffery, who had every qualification and diploma in the book, both surgical and medical, as an expert witness, was the wizard of the witness stand. He was able to build anything from a car to an electronic organ and used to make working models of bones and joints and demonstrate them to the court. I'm not sure if the judge really liked this because everyone got carried away with what amounted to a fascinating lecture by Jeff, and the actual case somehow seemed to get lost.

When giving expert evidence on oath one has to have all one's wits about one. It has always seemed unfair to me that one cannot ask questions back, or argue a point with Counsel. But that is the way the law works and quite correctly strict rules of evidence have to be obeyed.

In November 1972 Rita Hayworth was over here making a film and caught a bad cold and cough. She was off shooting for a week or more. The doctors looking after her then proposed she should have much more time off to recuperate.

I was engaged by the insurers to investigate the matter, but in the circumstances I felt a senior consultant physician of great experience should see her first and give his opinion before I dealt strictly with the insurance side. Her continued absence from the studios was running up a sizeable claim, and the production company and the insurers were getting very worried.

The result was a joint examination at the Dorchester Hotel between one of her doctors, the consultant and myself in Miss Hayworth's suite. As is the custom the three of us went up in the lift but no discussion of the case took place, and simple pleasantries were exchanged.

We were ushered through the living room into Miss Hayworth's bedroom. She was sitting on her bed in a negligee ready for the examination. She was tense, her beautiful eyes wide and staring. In order to save her any undue distress it was agreed that Dr. Dow alone should examine her and we should accept his findings.

I watched her submit to his various tests. When Dr. Dow told her kindly she had made a good recovery, it was as though she had been told the opposite. She sprang to her feet and stalked up and down claiming that she was not recovered and was not well enough to film. Tears began to stream down those beautiful high-boned cheeks; tears of anger and frustration.

To see this beautiful idol of mine in such a state was particularly shocking to me. I had been so utterly entranced by her in the past, seeing her as the incarnation of glamour, and now that illusion had been destroyed.

Now she raged about the conditions in which she had to work, and the cold and the rain which she had been subjected to as the cause of her present state. She screamed at us as though we were tormenters come to increase her misery. No reassurances on our part could calm her. She ordered us out of her room. Under this attack the doctors retreated. No sooner had we exited than she burst through the elegant double doors and asked us to wait. Sobbing she apologized for being so aggressive. It was a scene I suppose which must have been repeated in similar situations throughout pictures all over the world – the case of the star who had lost her confidence. In the English studios she had not received the respect, cosseting, and adulation she had been used to. The years had passed and the adoring cocooning world she had known as a great star was no longer there. It was removed on her first day of shooting. A chance remark by a young member of the production team on the set had upset her terribly. It was 'Who's Rita Hayworth?'

In my whole experience I had never felt less like performing the job I had to do. But the hard facts of the situation had to be assessed. I was a doctor and medically she was physically fit, and there were no signs of mental illness. Neither Dr. Dow nor myself could find any substance for a continuing medical claim. In the end Miss Hayworth, defeated, agreed, if the conditions of work could be changed, then she could film. Temperament, anguish and dissatisfaction with conditions of work were not medical grounds. There was a difference of medical opinion from her doctor.

Sadly I reported my view to the insurers who were waiting downstairs in the foyer, as I wrote later in my report.

'Emotionally she has become sufficiently upset now to produce temperamental outbursts, of which she gave ample demonstration during my interview with her. She appears very worried that things have gone unhappily for her in this film – that is to say, the bad luck of getting a virus infection, which she attributes wholly to the conditions under which she had to work. My talk with her and observation of her behaviour do not, however, lead me to believe that she is suffering from any underlying mental illness which would require special treatment by a psychiatrist, or which would prevent her in fact from resuming work. She fears, however, that the same conditions could make her ill again.

'In my view, reassurance by the production company that on resumption of work she would not be subjected to any wet, cold or unduly chilling conditions, combined with medication for a good night's sleep, and the development around her of a general atmosphere of encouragement and calm, should be sufficient to restore her confidence and emotional composure. Indeed, I feel that resumption of work would be the best therapeutic aid to such an outcome.'

A call was put out for Miss Hayworth to go to the studios and resume work. But she did not put in an appearance, and it transpired that she had left the country and flown back to the States. I could understand her action but the film company understandably sued her for breach of contract.

The case came up for hearing in the Superior Court of the State of California for the County of Los Angeles in 1973. I was told I would be required to give evidence there. I could get no assurance as to how long the case would last. It seemed I might be over the pond for weeks. I wondered what would be left of my practice when I returned. My solicitor advised me not to leave England. As a consequence I gave evidence under oath in the American Embassy in London before the Vice-Consul, Counsel for Miss Hayworth, the defendant, and Counsel for the film company, the plaintiff. These people had flown over to London to take witnesses' testimony. Before I gave evidence I obtained a signed letter from Miss Hayworth that she would not make any claim whatsoever against me on giving evidence or disclosing medical documents and records relating to her medical history.

On 25 January 1974 I remember being conducted down some long corridors in the embassy feeling some apprehension especially as at one or two corners well-lit portraits of Richard Nixon looked me straight in the eye.

It was a small room and we sat in comfortable chairs, but it was a court of law none the less, and technically at least I was in a foreign country. All the evidence was taken down in shorthand. I was sworn in in front of the Vice-Consul who was presiding and the questioning began.

Only those who have had to give evidence in a court will appreciate the strangely intimidating effect which the panoply and majesty of the legal process can evoke. Although as an expert witness, one is there to help the court to reach a just verdict, and is not there for anything oneself has done, nor is one being accused of any act, the uneasy feeling remains that somehow one is on trial for something. Even the opening routine questions sound sinister.

The two Counsels start to attack each other with words, words, words. As I remember it the opposing Counsel interjected with a complicated statement something like this. 'Before the doctor answers I must respectfully object to the question on several grounds. First and foremost the hypothetical question is not stated in any manner which the doctor can reasonably answer because the conditions have not been established with reasonable certainty as to the hypothetical question; secondly there is not sufficient background laid as to the expertise specially required for this kind of estimate by the doctor; and thirdly the question is so complex that if the additional elements which are required were to be supplied, it would be unable to be answered in one single question.'

My Counsel carries on.

'Let me ask you first, Doctor, do you remember the question I put to you?'

'Yes.'

'Do you understand the question I put to you?'

'Yes.'

'Do you find it too complex to answer?'

'No.'

'You can answer the question.'

The cross examination is usually the tough one. It is a question largely of evading traps which one has to see in advance. Mine ended, 'Your sole reason for being there was to evaluate the physical condition for insurance purposes only?'

'Not just physical, no.'

'The entire condition.'

'The medical condition.'

'For insurance purposes only?'

'Yes.'

'Thank you. I have nothing further.'

The re-examination elucidates points which may still be unclear. My Counsel concluded, 'Finally, could you distinguish for me between one's medical well-being as opposed to one's physical well-being?'

'The phrase "medical well-being" includes physical and mental.'

'And that is the distinction?'

'The distinction . . .'

'The "medical" encompasses the two?'

'Certainly.'

'I have no further questions. Thank you very much, Dr. Thorn.'

And my ordeal was over. I don't know what evidence Dr. Dow gave but he said to me in his Scottish accent afterwards,

'Another time laddie, if it's one of these film affairs, include me out.'

The case was finally settled in California. I have no idea what terms were agreed.

After the hearing, I went back home and had a lovely cup of Indian tea.

18 Over-Exposure

It has been said that the greatest pleasures of life are concerned with the filling or emptying of a hollow viscus. On a physiological level there is much going for this idea. To hold the mouth full of a vintage claret at its prime for one red velvety second before allowing it to be taken on the flood, out of control down the oesophagus; to empty the rectum quietly after breakfast while reading *The Times*; to discharge the contents of the seminal vesicles into the Pouch of Douglas of one's beloved, are all pleasures few would gainsay. But the emptying of the bladder has a quality of its own which sets its enjoyment from the others, being the only one where (for men at any rate) a visual bonus is provided.

No better example of the glorious varieties and components of the flashing stream – force, diameter, torque, or sheer parabolic virtuosity – was provided than at my first Merton College Gaudy.

The irresistible urge started during the last speech from High Table. The name of the torturer I have forgotten. We had passed the decanters several times, fiddled with the college silver, and shifted from buttock to buttock on the hard benches for what seemed an endless period.

'I fear I shall have to go,' I whispered to Mike Keating-Hill.

'So shall I,' he replied softly and then loudly said 'Hear Hear', directing these words at the speaker quite without any suitable context.

'Steady as she goes boys,' warned Harry Slater looking up towards High Table. 'I have the impression that our long-winded friend has got the message himself.'

It was at this point that we heard from the opposite side of the hall a pair of shoes treading stealthily over the creaking boards. The first stricken Mertonian made a rapid exit from the hall. With hardly a second's break another pair of footsteps started from our side, then two others and then in groups of twos and fours at varying speeds and with variable dignity, the long room echoed with the hollow sounds of retreating footsteps. Abruptly the speaker wound up, offered a final hurried toast and then sat down.

'OK,' said Harry, 'now.'

We rose as one man. Gaderene-like, nearly all the guests raced in unseemly haste towards the end of the hall, and squeezed through the narrow oak doorway. Down the stone steps three at a time, round to the left and under the archway. Finally into the haven of the smallest and oldest college quadrangle in Europe, burst a desperate rabble of old, middle-aged, and young sometime undergraduates.

Spaced in an imperfect circle round mob quad, from the wearers of all those learned gowns, those black or white ties, those decorations, medals and honours, shimmering in the moonlight, rose a veritable floribunda, a hissing academic cascade which fell on to the greensward. The sigh of consummate relief which followed wafted away to mingle with the sound of falling leaves in the avenue of limes in the Fellows' garden.

Shortly after the war, long before the College Gaudy, the same Mike Keating-Hill was staying with a fellow Mertonian, Maurice Hodgson, having been allowed to sleep for the night on the living-room couch by Hodge's wife Norma. The reason why even the murmur of the name Keating-Hill used to induce a Pavlovian rage in Norma for the next twenty years was because Mike failed to learn the geography of the house. Waking in the small hours with an imperative need, sleepily he gave up the search too easily and used a large Chinese vase standing on a plinth in the corner. He was not to know (and Norma was only to find out what use he had made of it after he had left), that the vase was where she kept her knitting.

For the first night of *Taking Things Quietly* at Malvern, I sat in the traditional author's box which was at one side of the dress-circle. With me was a suitably glamorous companion. Such was the odd geography of the theatre that the only way to get from the box to the loos was to walk across the dress-circle in front of the first row of seats, to the exit on the other side. Almost as we sat down the curtain went up on the first act. Half-way through it, there comes a tense moment in the plot when the stage is empty and the audience is in anticipatory silence. Then Sid Gullet the aged burglar climbs through a window of the barrister's home and begins an inspection to see if there is any silver or other valuables lying about. At the beginning of this silence my companion whispered to me,

'I shall have to go to the loo.'

'What?' I said, half attentive, my eyes fixed on the stage, gratified that the audience were reacting exactly as I wanted – in expectant silence.

'I've got to go to the loo,' she repeated and stood up.

'What on earth are you doing?' I hissed. 'Sit down.'

'Didn't you hear me?.'

'Will you please shut up and sit down.'

'If I don't go, I shall burst.'

'You can't go now.'

'I've got to . . . I'm sorry . . .'

She made a move towards the door of the box. I put out a restraining arm.

'You can't walk across the front of the dress circle . . .' I spluttered. 'It'll wreck the whole scene.'

'Don't worry, I'll duck down.'

'You're crazy,' I said frantically, 'I'm not having my play ruined by you causing a disturbance just at this moment . . . on the first night . . . you'll have to hold it . . .'

'I shall burst . . . I've told you.'

'Then burst in the back of the box,' I said desperately.

'Right,' she replied at the back of the box. 'If that's how you want it . . .'

Suddenly, what seemed to me with deafening sibilance, the hiss of a stream of water which would not have disgraced a young mare, came from behind me. I looked round to see my playmate squatting with a smile of profound relief on her face, as she urinated on to the dark red Wilton. A roar of laughter from the audience gave me one of the most acutely embarrassing moments of my life. Then I realized it was Sid Gullet's demonstration on the other side of the footlights that had evoked the mirth, not the performance behind me. There was a short burst of spontaneous applause. With astounding aplomb my girl-friend pulled up her panties, pushed down her skirt, sat in her chair again, and undaunted, clapped her hands with the rest. Sweating, I smiled with sickly pride into the auditorium.

The immediate crisis had been averted but I felt uneasy as our shoes made squelching sounds when we left the box in the first interval.

I slept fitfully that night in the hotel. Roy Limbert, who owned the theatre, was obsessively proud of its sparkle and polish. I didn't know how I could face him the next day, unless I could disguise the awful state of the carpet in the box I had occupied. I envisaged worse than that. In my half-sleeping state I saw stains appearing on the ceiling over the stalls underneath.

I got up at six and went down to the theatre. Everything was locked up of course. Just before seven the cleaning women arrived. I followed them in stealthily, and lurked about. At length one went to clean the fateful box. She entered it with her Hoover and switched on the light and the motor. Perhaps it had all dried up and nothing would be noticed. But after a few seconds the machine stopped. She leant over the box rail and called down to her companion working in the stalls below. 'Beryl?'

'Yes?'

'Come up here a minute, will you?'

'What's up?'

'I want you to look at something.'

Beryl, puffing noisily, eventually climbed up to the circle and went into the box.

I listened from behind a pillar a few yards away.

'Well, there are no water pipes long 'ere,' I heard clearly.

'No . . .'

There was a pause.

'Can you smell anything?'

'Yes . . .'

There was another pause.

'Well, I never . . .'

'It couldn't be that . . .'

'It could . . .'

'I know . . .'

'What . . .'

'A cat's done it. That's what it is.'

I felt there was some truth in the remark. I crept away, and later in the day, like a coward, drove my companion back to London, not daring to have a meeting with either Roy Limbert or E.P. Clift of the management. At the end of the week, I went back to Malvern again on my own. I furtively inspected the carpet in the box. There was a decidedly light patch visible in one corner. For all I know there probably still is. I sat in the stalls. The play seemed to be settling down nicely.

The pleasures of urination and the humorous aspects of it have been noted since time immemorial. Stories are widespread through the literature of all languages. It rapidly becomes a subject of fascination to young children. My own favourite of this era I found depicted in a charming French print which I first came across in the loo of a restaurant called Casa Comminetti in Lewisham some years ago. There is a prettily dressed little girl of about six pushing her doll's pram in the park. She has stopped to look round at a small boy of the same age wearing short trousers who is peeing against a tree-trunk. The caption is delightful, *'C'est vraiment commode, ça!'* Useful indeed. The picture hinted at the French genius for diplomacy, and reminded me of the World War II joke where the American G.I., performing in a *pissoir* in Paris, wanted to know the time. He enquired of the Frenchman at his side with the question 'Say, bo . . .?' After a quick glance of appraisal, the reply came back *'Oui monsieur. C'est magnifique!'*

The euphemisms for urination, including the official medical *micturition*, are legion, and we all have our favourites. The word is often a pointer to the character and age of the user. My uncle Jeff always enquired if one wanted to squeeze a lemon. He once considered being a fruit grower in South Africa but ended up managing a shipping firm in Takoradi. My uncle Morris Fox always 'went for a leak'. Incidentally, his invitation to a meal was invariably phrased 'Shall we graze?' Needless to say, he was a farmer. He used to live rather comfortably at Potters Marston Hall. My father, who could reduce any idea to an algebraical formula, regarded a drink as a plus and a pee as a minus, the 'p' he would observe to captive junior classes, being silent as in swimming. Uncle Charlie, his younger brother, always had a 'Jimmy Riddle' and Uncle Jack Fox, who was the colonel of his regiment and was awarded an M.C. in World War I, always went to 'shake hands with an old friend'.

The vicar at Barrow-on-Soar transmuted the subject into one of divine dispensation. When little May Southwark, overcome by the Bishop's presence at her confirmation, left a trail all down the aisle, the reverend parish incumbent raised his eyes heavenwards and remarked, 'Ah me. The roof again.' This in spite of a long spell of fine summer weather.

My uncle Fred, a headmaster like my father, never referred to the activity at all.

At Shrewsbury we used the word 'pump' and one pumped into one's handleless 'gerry'. Once lights were out the bedroom monitor was a complete dictator, benevolent or otherwise. Permission had to be obtained from him to 'blow' or 'pump'. Some monitors used sanctions unfairly and invented rules for their special amusement. I cannot remember now whether it was Denys Johnson or George (Bellclapper) Bruckshaw who each night for several weeks had to kneel before Richard Hillary holding the gerry on top of his own head and respectfully make the request, 'Please pump, Oh King,' and remain in position regardless of any wavering aim from above. Recalled in retrospect down the long corridor of the years, this ritualistic barbarism seems incredible.

There were of course reprisals against the monitors which I, being on the science side, was pressed upon by my classical contemporaries, to provide. A tiny crystal of potassium permanganate will colour pints of urine an unhealthy blood-red and can lead to a horrid shock in the morning and a conviction that haemorrhage has struck in the night. More dramatic and more dangerous is to place in the receptacle a small piece of metallic sodium which, as every schoolboy knows, reacts violently on contact with water. It may have been Pitcairn-Campbell or Chappel-Gill who lost his 'bush' for a while in this manner, but I cannot be sure.

I was, however, to be reminded of the crackle and smell of scorching pubic hair a few years later as a medical student at the Radcliffe Infirmary. The professor of obstetrics and gynaecology was demonstrating to a group of us how to cauterize a cervical erosion. The lower half of the patient was exposed in the traditional lithotomy position. She was a placid woman of about thirty and her view of us was suitably screened off.

A probationary nurse was asked by the Prof. to swab the vagina and cervix with a Flavine solution. This the girl did with a long pair of forceps carrying a piece of cotton wool dipped in the yellow fluid. A strong light shone up the Cusco's speculum for us all to stare and wonder.

As he took hold of the instrument, the Professor peeped over the screen and reassured the patient, using his carefully modulated and refined Scottish accent.

'Now, my dear, this won't hurrrt at all.'

'I know doctor,' came the reply.

'You can trust me absolutely.'

As the red hot end of the cautery instrument probed up the vagina for the erosion, the surgeon's words were shown to be a vile falsehood. A blue flash shot out from the unimaginable depths. To me, the familiar crackle of burning pubic hair followed. After a moment of stunned silence there was a general collapse into uncontrolled laughter of all of us except the nurse, the patient and the Prof. His expression was first astonished, and then livid. He snatched up the pot of Flavine and sniffed it. Rounding on the nurse, he barked, 'You cretinous idiot! You've used Flavine in spirit instead of the aqueous solution!'

The nurse dissolved into tears, but our teacher quickly regained his style and dignity. He looked over the screen and said to the patient reassuringly, 'There now, that didn't hurrrt, did it?'

'Oh no, doctor,' came the confident reply, 'It just felt warm, that's all.'

Physiologically, urination is achieved through the pathway of the pelvic nerves, the sacral nerves, the hypogastric ganglia, and centres in the spinal cord, mid-brain and hind-brain. The mechanism is complex. The higher centres of the brain, and indeed the personality of the individual, play an enormous part. Suggestion, both for initiation or inhibition of the flashing stream is often the deciding factor. In my patients' lavatory in Harley Street hangs a watercolour I painted many years ago of a waterfall at Buxton, itself famous for its water. The idea is that the picture will act as a psychological diuretic. A specimen required for testing is not such an easy thing to obtain as one might suppose. Some patients develop an uncanny knack of having just 'been' before an examination; others find it impossible to let go. I find a useful way of persuading a tense patient to pass water is to give the useful advice to sing, whistle or run the taps in the basin, and then add, 'If you can't, it doesn't matter.' This throw-away attitude reduces inhibition, and often does the trick. To the plea 'There isn't any there, doctor', it can always be pointed out that the kidneys are making urine all the time. Of course there is no reply to the laughing statement made by a West Indian patient after a ten minute attempt: 'He don't want to!'

I have had to collect specimens and test the urines of many people for insurance purposes, in many different places and circumstances. There have been some memorable incidents, amongst the film artistes. The receptacle itself has often provided a subject of interest. When I flew to Rhodes to examine the cast of the first make of *The Guns of Navarone* in 1960, I had warned the production manager that I would need some receptacle for the collection of urine. I wasn't going to take a glass vessel by air a thousand miles or more for this simple procedure. When I reached the hotel where the film unit was based, I accepted the tumbler which was given me for the purpose.

'I can't ask the ladies to pee into this,' I exclaimed. 'OK for Gregory Peck and David Niven, but I'll need something wider and bigger for the girls.'

The local assistant made a gesture of complete comprehension and left the room where I was to do the examinations. Shortly afterwards a waiter returned with a beautiful cut-glass salad bowl which was prettily made use of by Maria Papas.

Some years later I used to take a medium sized Woolworth's plastic mixing bowl in my bag for lightness' sake, for examinations outside my consulting room. I was charmed when Marlene Dietrich having obliged in her suite at the Savoy, took a great interest in the simple use of a test dipstick for albumin and sugar. After I had rinsed and washed the bowl, she insisted on personally cleaning it meticulously and drying it for me to return to my bag.

A doctor, like a mother-in-law, is frequently presented as a comic music-hall figure, and medical examination jokes are legion, including the masterpiece about the blood-donor as portrayed by Tony Hancock (whom I examined without incident of any sort in 1964). Actors, being by calling inventive and imaginative, are not averse to playing tricks on the medical examiner.

In the early sixties I had to examine a prestigious cast for an international production. Appointments were made at twenty minute intervals, and near the end of the session six urine glasses stood labelled and ready for testing on the lavatory shelf. The last to come was Trevor Howard.

About six months later Trevor (whom I came to know well over the years) had to be seen before he made another film. As he was about to leave, he asked me with his misleadingly innocent smile, how his urine was the last time? I looked up the card.

'Fine,' I said. 'Quite normal, why do you ask?'

'Well, doc,' he grinned, 'I have a confession to make. The last time I was here I couldn't do any, so I put a little urine from all the other glasses into mine.'

When we had stopped laughing, I said, 'How lucky for you that Ingrid Bergman wasn't pregnant.'

Through an oversight, which at one time was not infrequent, the cast of the musical *One Step into Spring* had not been insured, even by the day before shooting. Panic medicals were requested. I went to the Dorchester where the rehearsals were going on next to the Orchid Room. Time was of the essence. I filled in the question-form sitting at a table which was being laid by hotel staff for an evening banquet. The young man I was examining – Leo Sayer – stripped to the waist without embarrassment, and I completed the physical while the work went on around us. The question of the urine test then arose. As it happened I had no collecting bottle with me. Remembering the Isle of Rhodes technique I approached an elderly waiter and explained my dilemma. He disappeared, and returned, with a wine-glass on a tray. He checked it for cleanliness and give it a professional polish before offering it to me. Leo retired to a corner of the room, performed in the glass and brought it back to me. I tested the fluid while Leo put the glass back on the waiter's tray. The latter bowed and went out of the room. Not a word had been spoken, not an expression had flitted across his features. Jeeves could not have done us more proud.

The spontaneous witticisms of the Master are in large measure apocryphal, but Mr. Coward's comment in his suite at the Savoy should be recorded: having concluded the examination, I asked him if he could produce a specimen.

'I'm not at all sure about that dear boy,' he said.

By way of encouragement I answered, 'I only need a teaspoonful.'

'I don't happen to have a teaspoon,' was the clipped reply.

Very recently an old friend of mine, Oliver Reed, came to be examined for the film *Christopher Columbus*. I told him I was writing a light hearted autobiography and asked him if he had had any amusing medical experiences. He thought a moment and then laughed.

'Yes, I've got one for you. Something that happened to me one night.'

'What was that?' I asked.

Oliver told me that one Christmas Eve in Los Angeles he and a friend made it a champagne evening, to such a degree that Oliver suddenly decided he would like two eagle's claws tattooed on his 'knob' as he put it.

A visit to several of the more orthodox practitioners of the art met with flat refusals. The cab driver came to the rescue.

'I know who'll do it,' he said.

'Then take me there, my good fellow,' said Oliver.

They weaved through the somewhat rough Mexican quarter of the city. The cab stopped and Oliver mounted the stairs where two Koreans, a man and his wife were both tattooists. The man shook his head, but his wife was made of sterner stuff. She led Mr. Reed through a beaded screen and performed the job to satisfaction.

'May I have a look?' I asked him.

'Be my guest.'

Two exquisitely executed claws adorned the end of his member.

When we had stopped laughing, I said, 'I can't put that in my book.'

'Why on earth not?' asked Oliver.

'But surely you don't want everyone who reads the book to know about it?'

'What's it matter about them? All my friends know, naturally.'

'I realize that,' I said, 'but you might change your mind and then sue me for . . .'

'Don't be so distrustful, Ronnie. You can put it in, I tell you. I'll sign a thing giving you permission here and now if you like.'

'Well,' I said cautiously. 'You'd better think about it. See how it looks written down. I'll send it to you, then if you still don't mind you can give me written permission to publish it.'

'Of course,' he said. 'But there's another bit to the story.' He still had his shirt off for the medical and pointed to his left shoulder. 'You've noticed this because you once mentioned it.'

Over his deltoid was a neatly tattooed eagle's head. I murmured my admiration. Oliver grinned broadly.

'You see, when people say "Why, you've got an Eagle's head on your shoulder," I then reply, "Would you like to see where it's perched?"'

19 'Forthcoming Attractions'

Before I went under the anaesthetic for my hip replacement operation at Charing Cross Hospital in May 1981 I kept muttering 'De profundis, de profundis'. I think the nurses whose voices had the varied accents of the earth in them – the dear earth I was about to leave – Indian, Malaysian, Jamaican, Chinese, thought I was asking for food or water because they patiently explained I could not have anything by mouth now that I was on my pre-med.

I thought about the last six months, in which my world seemed to have fallen apart. During the mid-week at the end of January, Halina had gone down to the cottage as she often did while I finished my stint in the 'Strasse' to join her at the weekend. As I was about to open the flat door to leave for Harley Street, an envelope came through the letter-box. I opened it and took out the letter. It was from her solicitors. They informed me succinctly that my wife had gone to Burford and I was not to follow her. Moreover, I was not to attempt to see her, or get in touch with her by letter or telephone. If I did, a court order restraining me would be applied for. They went on to say that settlement of all property, furniture and belongings was to be made in due course.

I stood quite still and read the document through three times. We had had our differences and quarrels, who hasn't? But that letter hit me like a missile. I went into the bedroom and opened her wardrobes. Yes, it was true. Her clothes had gone. The sight of empty coathangers can be sickeningly macabre. I looked round the flat and for the first time noticed other things were not in their usual places. Confused, my mind teeming with questions, I put the letter in my pocket and went to see my day's patients. When I came back in the evening I sat in my chair, sat and thought into the night. Eventually sleep overtook me. Lily Harris our housekeeper found me unshaven and still in my crumpled clothes. She made my breakfast as usual. And then I asked her a question I had never asked her before.

'Have you a cigarette by any chance, Lily?'

'Yes, doctor,' she replied, surprised, and gave me one. It seemed the time was ripe to start the old habit, as Count Basie would say, one more once.

All my attempts at reconciliation failed and eventually I was forced to seek a divorce from Halina. Anyone who has been through this hurtful and shattering business with all its petty details and to-ing and fro-ing about small worthless objects knows how awful it can be. Now it is all over I can say I harbour no malice, but not then, not then, not as I lay in the hard hospital bed waiting to go into the theatre for John Strachan and Lippy-Kessel to exercise their skill and care upon my long-suffering and hated hip-joint. I had lost my cottage, and even my flat was under attack; my financial resources were small and inadequate. I was worried that my absence from the practice for the operation would prejudice its future. My secretary Angela Smith was holding it all together with tact and devotion, but for how long, how long? My real assets were just me, my dear daughters and my skills. But my spirit was very low and I questioned my ability or even desire to exercise them again. I was so tired of it all. I didn't think I had the energy to struggle any more. I was afraid and lonely. As the nurse put the needle in my arm and drowsiness came upon me, I prayed – something I had not done for many a year. The prayer was a simple one. 'Dear God, please don't let me survive this operation.'

I learnt later that I very nearly didn't, but in the end the replacement was a huge success. To be free of pain, and able to move about as I hadn't moved for years; to throw away my stick and my limp and escape the tyranny of pain-relieving drugs was like a rejuvenation. I felt twenty years younger, and gradually, I'm told, I began to look it. My practice did not collapse, indeed it seemed to thrive anew, under June Horsley's devoted attentions.

I realized after the first muzzy days following the operation that I was, after all, going to survive. The first faces I recognized smiling at me mistily were those of Ted Eveleigh and Denys Johnson, Roger Frisby and Deirdre, of my daughter Vanessa and my son-in-law, Richard Fergusson. With growing strength I lost my self-pity and despair. I was rich beyond compare. As the gifts and cards and the flowers came in, and then the phone-calls, I realized I never knew how many friends and acquaintances I had collected. It was a revelation. Who were all these well-wishers I had neglected? I began to take a different view of things. Could it possibly be that my accountant, David Ufland, and my bank manager, John Mellers, really cared about me? Yes they did, as I have confirmed long since.

Amanda came over from San Francisco leaving her husband, Richard Rumble, in order to get me out of hospital. Thelma and Raymond, and the Fergussons rallied round. I reached the stage where I could run if not jump, and went back to Harley Street on springy feet and with equal length legs.

I suppose by the autumn of that year the thought was growing at the back of my mind that perhaps now was the time to write my autobiography. At least I could put my experiences down. Yet is was not about me I wanted to talk. It was about all the people I had met and knew and remembered. I thought of all those that I had not seen for years – my oldest friend Philip Whitfield living in Vancouver; my cousin June who had trod the boards in many a repertory threatre; my cousin Doreen and her brother Bobby and his seven sons. Where were they all now?

And as I thought about my life, largely spent examining litigants and film artistes – all those thousands of stars who had given pleasure to so many – it seemed as though I was suddenly in the midst of a familiar crowd. Those that had passed away still lived on with me in my memory. Perhaps I could record something of their personalities for others to share.

When my friends Richie and Carolee Bradshaw, who live in Manhattan Beach, Beverly Hills, took me round to the empty lots and sets still standing at Twentieth Century-Fox and MGM, I imaged I saw ghosts of people I had known, and heard familiar voices. I decided to write about them all.

But I don't think I should really have started this book had I not gone to a small dinner party in a house behind Park Lane.

It was a mild evening and there were french windows. As I stood – now painlessly – drinking my Bloody Mary and listening to some jazz which was more than nostalgic, she came in through the windows – just like Elvira in *Blithe Spirit*. But her name was Muriel. I was immediately captivated. She was scintillating, glamorous, independent, witty. I learnt later she was a head-mistress; and a lot later, the sweetest kindest woman I have ever known.

'Hello,' I said. 'Where have you come from?'

'Out there,' she waved a slender arm. 'Isn't it a wonderful evening?'

'I hadn't paid much attention to it until this moment.'

'Well please come on the balcony and look,' she commanded.

Muriel took my hand and I followed. I could see the familiar trees of Berkeley Square in the distance. The lights were twinkling everywhere. I took a deep breath of the October air.

'Well?' she asked.

'So *this* is Mayfair!' I exclaimed.

'As if you didn't know.'

She produced a deep gurgle. Much more of this and I knew I was a goner. And there was much much more. She was a beautiful perfectly proportioned blonde. All my life I thought, I have been falling for sultry brunettes and all the time, I knew at that instant, what I had wanted, what I had really been searching for was a bubbly sexy blonde. And this was the blonde I knew I was going to marry.

As we sat at the table throughout the meal I probably overdid the verbal entertainment. What Muriel said so perceptively watered the seed that has become this book.

'Quite a little raconteur, aren't you?' she remarked.

'I like to think so,' was my reply.

THE BEGINNING

Index

The author would like to apologize to all the 6,000 or so artistes he has examined who are not included in this index for reasons of space. Only those referred to in the text are listed.

173